The Guide to Clinical Preventive Services

2012

Recommendations of the U.S. Preventive Services Task Force

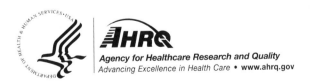

AHRQ
Agency for Healthcare Research and Quality
Advancing Excellence in Health Care • **www.ahrq.gov**

The clinical summaries in the *Guide* are abridged versions of recommendations from the U.S. Preventive Services Task Force (USPSTF). To view the full recommendation statements, supporting evidence, or recommendations published after March 2012, go to www.USPreventiveServicesTaskForce.org.

The USPSTF Electronic Preventive Services Selector (ePSS) allows users to download the USPSTF recommendations to PDA, mobile, or tablet devices; receive notifications of updates; and search and browse recommendations online. Users can search the ePSS for recommendations by patient age, sex, and pregnancy status. To download, subscribe, or search, go to www.epss.ahrq.gov.

Recommendations made by the USPSTF are independent of the U.S. Government. They should not be construed as an official position of AHRQ or the U.S. Department of Health and Human Services.

Foreword

Since 1998, the Agency for Healthcare Research and Quality (AHRQ) has convened the U.S. Preventive Services Task Force (USPSTF)—an independent panel of non-Federal experts in prevention and primary care. AHRQ staff provide scientific, technical, and administrative support for the Task Force, and assist in disseminating its findings and recommendations to key audiences.

In that role, we are pleased to make *The Guide to Clinical Preventive Services 2012* available to those who seek to ensure that their patients receive the highest quality clinical preventive services. Previous iterations of the USPSTF *Guide to Clinical Preventive Services* are used around the Nation to provide appropriate and effective preventive care.

This year's *Guide* includes some changes that will make it more user-friendly for practicing clinicians. The *Guide* comprises 64 preventive services, which now are presented in an easy-to-use, one-page summary table format. In addition, the *Guide* provides information on resources that clinicians can use to educate their patients on appropriate preventive services, as well as brief descriptions of and links to tools that they can use to improve their practices, including the electronic Preventive Services Selector, MyHealthfinder, and the Guide to Community Preventive Services (for more details, see Appendixes D and E).

As more information becomes available to clinicians and patients alike, AHRQ's goal is to help improve patients' health and well being, and contribute to better health outcomes for the Nation overall.

Carolyn M. Clancy, M.D.
Director
Agency for Healthcare Research and Quality

Preface

Since being codified by Congress, the U.S. Preventive Services Task Force (USPSTF) has been fulfilling its charge to conduct rigorous reviews of scientific evidence to create evidence-based recommendations for preventive services that should be provided in the primary care setting.

Since its inception, the USPSTF has made and maintained recommendations on more than 100 clinical preventive services that are intended to prevent or reduce the risk for heart disease, cancer, infectious diseases, and other conditions and events that impact the health of children, adolescents, adults, and pregnant women. The *Guide to Clinical Preventive Services 2012* includes new or updated recommendations on 64 clinical preventive services released from 2002-2012 in a brief, easily usable format meant for use at the point of patient care. Recommendations that were being updated while this edition of the *Guide* was being compiled, as well as the complete USPSTF recommendation statements, are available along with their supporting scientific evidence at www.USPreventiveServicesTaskForce.org.

Recommendations for preventive care have evolved over time. The suggestion that it is not beneficial to provide all of the services available for prevention was nearly a heretical concept in U.S. medical practice when the first USPSTF started its work. Over time, individual health care providers, professional organizations, integrated health systems, health plans and insurers, and public programs, including the Centers for Medicare & Medicaid Services as well as groups crafting health quality measures and national health objectives, have adopted the recommendations. The primary audience for the USPSTF's work remains primary care clinicians, and the recommendations are now considered by many to provide definitive standards for preventive services.

The work of the USPSTF is central to the preventive benefits covered under the Patient Protection and Affordable Care Act. Under the new law, in new plans and policies preventive services with a Task Force grade of A or B will be covered with no cost sharing requirements. Even prior to national reform activities, the USPSTF had increased the transparency of its work, and these efforts have gained additional momentum in view of the enhanced importance of the recommendations under the new law. Public comments are welcomed at multiple points in the development of each recommendation to allow for additional input from experts and advocates and to assist us in better crafting messages for the public. However, the USPSTF remains committed to evaluating evidence free from the influence of politics, special interests, and advocacy.

Our methods continue to evolve as well. Our Procedure Manual, which can be found at www.USPreventiveServicesTaskForce.org/uspstf08/methods/procmanual. htm, outlines our updated process for evaluating the quality and strength of the evidence for a service, determining the net health benefit (benefits minus harms) associated with the service, and judging the level of certainty that providing these services will be beneficial in primary care. We continue to explore the appropriate use of mathematical modeling to help fill research gaps regarding the ages at which to start and stop providing a service, and at what time intervals. In addition, we are committed to improving the communication of our recommendations to a broader audience, including patients and policymakers.

As before, the letter grade linked to each recommendation reflects the magnitude of net benefit and the strength and certainty of the evidence supporting the provision of a specific preventive service. These grades translate to practice guidance for clinicians:

- Discuss services with "A" and "B" recommendations with eligible patients and offer them as a priority.

- Discourage the use of services with "D" recommendations unless there are unusual additional considerations.

- Give lower priority to services with "C" recommendations; they need not be provided unless there are individual considerations in favor of providing the service.

- Help patients understand the uncertainty surrounding services when the evidence is insufficient to determine net benefit (I statement). Clinicians may read the Clinical Considerations section of the full recommendations for additional guidance.

As is true of all patient care, preventive services have become much more complex in view of ongoing research. The USPSTF realizes that clinical decisions about patients involve more complex considerations than the evidence alone; clinicians should always understand the evidence but individualize decisionmaking to the specific patient and situation. While providers and patients look for simple messages and actions, our recommendations reflect the advances in knowledge in this critical area of health services, and, in order to maximize the health benefits and decrease any health harms, we must consider the new complexity as we do for all medical services we provide. The Clinical Considerations section of each USPSTF recommendation statement helps clinicians by offering practical information so they can tailor these recommendations to individual patients.

We strongly encourage clinicians to visit the USPSTF Web site and read the complete recommendation statements for those services they provide, as the additional information can help them deliver the highest quality preventive care. In addition, the USPSTF Electronic Preventive Services Selector (ePSS), available via PDA, smart phone, or on the Web at www.epss.ahrq.gov, allows users to search USPSTF recommendations by patient age and other clinical characteristics.

We hope you find the *Guide to Clinical Preventive Services 2012* to be a useful tool as you care for patients. Based on the best medical evidence available, we are confident that by implementing these recommended services, you will help your patients live longer and healthier lives.

Virginia A. Moyer, M.D., M.P.H., Chair
Michael L. LeFevre, M.D., M.S.P.H., Co-Vice Chair
Albert L. Siu, M.D., M.S.P.H., Co-Vice Chair
U.S. Preventive Services Task Force

Contents

Foreword...iii

Preface v

Preventive Services Recommended by the USPSTF 1

Recommendations for Adults (alphabetical list) 5

Abdominal Aortic Aneurysm, Screening...7
Alcohol Misuse, Screening and Behavioral Counseling...8
Aspirin for the Prevention of Cardiovascular Disease, Preventive Medication 9
Aspirin or NSAIDS for Prevention of Colorectal Cancer,
    Preventive Medication 10
Bacterial Vaginosis in Pregnancy, Screening 11
Bacteriuria, Screening..12
*Bladder Cancer, Screening 13
Breast and Ovarian Cancer, BRCA Testing, Screening..14
Breast Cancer, Screening 15, 16
Breastfeeding, Counseling 17
Carotid Artery Stenosis, Screening 18
*Cervical Cancer, Screening 19
Chlamydial Infection, Screening 20
Chronic Obstructive Pulmonary Disease, Screening...21
Colorectal Cancer, Screening...22
Coronary Heart Disease (Risk Assessment, Nontraditional Risk Factors),
    Screening...23
Depression in Adults, Screening 24
Diabetes Mellitus, Screening 25
Folic Acid Supplementation, Preventive Medication...26
Genital Herpes Simplex, Screening...27
Gestational Diabetes, Screening..28
Glaucoma, Screening...29
Gonorrhea, Screening..30
Hemochromatosis, Screening 31
Hepatitis B Virus Infection, Screening..32
Hepatitis B Virus Infection (Pregnant Women), Screening.................................33
Hepatitis C Virus Infection, Screening 34
High Blood Pressure in Adults, Screening...35
HIV Infection, Screening 36
Hormone Replacement Therapy, Preventive Medication 37
Illicit Drug Use, Screening 38
Impaired Visual Acuity in Older Adults, Screening 39
Lipid Disorders in Adults, Screening 40

Lung Cancer, Screening...41
Motor Vehicle Occupant Restraints, Counseling 42
Oral Cancer, Screening..43
*Osteoporosis, Screening...44
Ovarian Cancer, Screening 45
Pancreatic Cancer, Screening..46
Peripheral Arterial Disease, Screening...47
Rh (D) Incompatibility, Screening...48
Sexually Transmitted Infections, Counseling 49
Skin Cancer, Screening...50
Suicide Risk, Screening...51
Syphilis Infection, Screening 52
Syphilis (Pregnant Women), Screening...53
*Testicular Cancer, Screening 54
Thyroid Disease, Screening..55
Tobacco Use in Adults, Counseling and Intervention 56

Recommendations for Children and Adolescents (alphabetical list) 57

Blood Lead Levels in Childhood and Pregnancy, Screening............59
Congenital Hypothyroidism, Screening.......................................60
Developmental Dysplasia of the Hip, Screening............................61
*Gonococcal Ophthalmia Neonatorum, Preventive Medication.......62
Hearing Loss (Newborn), Screening..63
Hyperbilirubinemia in Infants, Screening....................................64
Iron Deficiency Anemia, Screening 65, 66
Lipid Disorders in Children, Screening..67
Major Depressive Disorder in Children and Adolescents, Screening.................68
Obesity in Children and Adolescents, Screening............................69
Phenylketonuria, Screening..70
Scoliosis in Adolescents (Idiopathic), Screening...........................71
Sickle Cell Disease, Screening...72
Speech and Language Delay, Screening...73
*Visual Impairment in Children Ages 1-5, Screening 74

Immunizations 75

Topics in Progress 79

Appendixes and Index... 83

Appendix A. How the U.S. Preventive Services Task Force Grades Its
    Recommendations...85
Appendix B. Members of the U.S. Preventive Services Task Force 2002-2012....88
Appendix C. Acknowledgements..91
Appendix D. About the U.S. Preventive Services Task Force............94
Appendix E. More Resources...97
Index. Recommendations, Cross-Referenced.................................101

*New recommendations released March 2010 to March 2012.

Preventive Services Recommended by the USPSTF

Section 1: Preventive Services Recommended by the USPSTF

The U.S. Preventive Services Task Force (USPSTF) recommends that clinicians discuss these preventive services with eligible patients and offer them as a priority. All these services have received an "A" or a "B" (recommended) grade from the Task Force. For definitions of all grades used by the USPSTF, see Appendix A (beginning on p. 85). Clinical summaries of recommendations for adults begin on p. 5. Clinical summaries of recommendations for children begin on p. 57.

Recommendation	Adults		Special Populations	
	Men	Women	Pregnant Women	Children
Abdominal Aortic Aneurysm, Screening[1]	✓			
Alcohol Misuse Screening and Behavioral Counseling Interventions	✓	✓	✓	
Aspirin for Prevention of Cardiovascular Disease[2]	✓	✓		
Asymptomatic Bacteriuria in Adults, Screening[3]		✓	✓	
Breast and Ovarian Cancer Susceptibility, Genetic Risk Assessment and BRCA Mutation Testing[4]		✓		
Breast Cancer, Screening[5]		✓		
Breastfeeding, Primary Care Interventions to Promote[6]		✓	✓	
Cervical Cancer, Screening[7]		✓		
Chlamydial Infection, Screening[8]		✓	✓	
Colorectal Cancer, Screening[9]	✓	✓		
Congenital Hypothyroidism, Screening[10]				✓
Depression in Adults, Screening[11]	✓	✓		
Diabetes Mellitus (Type 2) in Adults, Screening[12]	✓	✓		
Folic Acid to Prevent Neural Tube Defects[13]		✓	✓	
Gonococcal Ophthalmia Neonatorum, Preventive Medication[14]				✓

Section 1: Preventive Services Recommended by the USPSTF (continued)

Recommendation	Adults		Special Populations	
	Men	Women	Pregnant Women	Children
Gonorrhea, Screening[15]		✓	✓	
Hearing Loss in Newborns, Screening[16]				✓
Hepatitis B Virus in Pregnant Women, Screening[17]			✓	✓
High Blood Pressure (Adults), Screening	✓	✓		
HIV, Screening[18]	✓	✓	✓	✓
Iron Deficiency Anemia, Prevention[19]				✓
Iron Deficiency Anemia, Screening[20]			✓	
Lipid Disorders in Adults, Screening[21]	✓	✓		
Major Depressive Disorder in Children, Screening[22]				✓
Obesity in Children and Adolescents, Screening[23]				✓
Osteoporosis, Screening[24]		✓		
Phenylketonuria, Screening[25]				✓
Rh (D) Incompatibility, Screening[26]			✓	✓
Sexually Transmitted Infections, Counseling[27]	✓	✓		✓
Sickle Cell Disease, Screening[28]				✓
Syphilis Infection, Screening[29]	✓	✓		
Syphilis Infection in Pregnancy, Screening			✓	
Tobacco Use in Adults and Pregnant Women, Counseling[30]	✓	✓	✓	
Visual Impairment in Children Ages 1 to 5, Screening[31]				✓

[1] One-time screening by ultrasonography in men aged 65 to 75 who have ever smoked.

[2] When the potential harm of an increase in gastrointestinal hemorrhage is outweighed by a potential benefit of a reduction in myocardial infarctions (men aged 45-79 years) or in ischemic strokes (women aged 55-79 years).

[3] Pregnant women at 12-16 weeks gestation or at first prenatal visit, if later.

[4] Refer women whose family history is associated with an increased risk for deleterious mutations in BRCA1 or BRCA 2 genes for genetic counseling and evaluation for BRCA testing.

[5] Biennial screening mammography for women aged 50 to 74 years. Note: The Department of Health and Human Services, in implementing the Affordable Care Act, follows the 2002 USPSTF recommendation for screening mammography, with or without clinical breast examination, every 1-2 years for women aged 40 and older.

[6] Interventions during pregnancy and after birth to promote and support breastfeeding.

[7] Screen with cytology every 3 years (women ages 21 to 65) or co-test (cytology/HPV testing) every 5 years (women ages 30-65).

[8] Sexually active women 24 and younger and other asymptomatic women at increased risk for infection. Asymptomatic pregnant women 24 and younger and others at increased risk.

[9] Adults aged 50-75 using fecal occult blood testing, sigmoidoscopy, or colonoscopy.

[10] Newborns.

[11] When staff-assisted depression care supports are in place to assure accurate diagnosis, effective treatment, and followup.

[12] Asymptomatic adults with sustained blood pressure greater than 135/80 mg Hg.

[13] All women planning or capable of pregnancy take a daily supplement containing 0.4 to 0.8 mg (400 to 800 µg) of folic acid.

[14] Newborns.

[15] Sexually active women, including pregnant women 25 and younger, or at increased risk for infection.

[16] Newborns.

[17] Screen at first prenatal visit.

[18] All adolescents and adults and increased risk for HIV infection and all pregnant women.

[19] Routine iron supplementation for asymptomatic children aged 6 to 12 months who are at increased risk for iron deficiency anemia.

[20] Routine screening in asymptomatic pregnant women.

[21] Men aged 20-35 and women over age 20 who are at increased risk for coronary heart disease; all men aged 35 and older.

[22] Adolescents (age 12 to 18) when systems are in place to ensure accurate diagnosis, psychotherapy, and followup.

[23] Screen children aged 6 years and older; offer or refer for intensive counseling and behavioral interventions.

[24] Women aged 65 years and older and women under age 65 whose 10-year fracture risk is equal to or greater than that of a 65-year-old white woman without additional risk factors.

[25] Newborns.

[26] Blood typing and antibody testing at first pregnancy-related visit. Repeated antibody testing for unsensitized Rh (D)-negative women at 24-28 weeks gestation unless biological father is known to be Rh (D) negative.

[27] All sexually active adolescents and adults at increased risk for STIs.

[28] Newborns.

[29] Persons at increased risk.

[30] Ask all adults about tobacco use and provide tobacco cessation interventions for those who use tobacco; provide augmented, pregnancy-tailored counseling for those pregnant women who smoke.

[31] Screen children ages 3 to 5 years.

Recommendations
for Adults

SCREENING FOR ABDOMINAL AORTIC ANEURYSM

CLINICAL SUMMARY OF U.S. PREVENTIVE SERVICES TASK FORCE RECOMMENDATION

Population	Men ages 65 to 75 years who have ever smoked	Men ages 65 to 75 years who have never smoked	Women ages 65 to 75 years
Recommendation	Screen once for abdominal aortic aneurysm with ultrasonography. Grade: B	No recommendation for or against screening. Grade: C	Do not screen for abdominal aortic aneurysm. Grade: D
Risk Assessment	The major risk factors for abdominal aortic aneurysm include male sex, a history of ever smoking (defined as 100 cigarettes in a person's lifetime), and age of 65 years or older.		
Screening Tests	Screening abdominal ultrasonography is an accurate test when performed in a setting with adequate quality assurance (i.e., in an accredited facility with credentialed technologists). Abdominal palpation has poor accuracy and is not an adequate screening test.		
Timing of Screening	One-time screening to detect an abdominal aortic aneurysm using ultrasonography is sufficient. There is negligible health benefit in re-screening those who have normal aortic diameter on initial screening.		
Interventions	Open surgical repair of an aneurysm of at least 5.5 cm leads to decreased abdominal aortic aneurysm-related mortality in the long term; however, there are major harms associated with this procedure.		
Balance of Benefits and Harms	In men ages 65 to 75 years who have ever smoked, the benefits of screening for abdominal aortic aneurysm outweigh the harms.	In men ages 65 to 75 years who have never smoked, the balance between the benefits and harms of screening for abdominal aortic aneurysm is too close to make a general recommendation for this population.	The potential overall benefit of screening for abdominal aortic aneurysm among women ages 65 to 75 years is low because of the small number of abdominal aortic aneurysm-related deaths in this population and the harms associated with surgical repair.
Other Relevant USPSTF Recommendations	The USPSTF has made recommendations on screening for carotid artery stenosis, coronary heart disease, high blood pressure, lipid disorders, and peripheral arterial disease. These recommendations are available at http://www.uspreventiveservicestaskforce.org/.		

For a summary of the evidence systematically reviewed in making this recommendation, the full recommendation statement, and supporting documents, please go to http://www.uspreventiveservicestaskforce.org/.

SCREENING AND BEHAVIORAL COUNSELING INTERVENTIONS IN PRIMARY CARE TO REDUCE ALCOHOL MISUSE

CLINICAL SUMMARY OF U.S. PREVENTIVE SERVICES TASK FORCE RECOMMENDATION

Population	Adults, including pregnant women	Adolescents
Recommendation	Screen and provide behavioral counseling interventions to reduce alcohol misuse. Grade: B	No recommendation. Grade: I (Insufficient Evidence)

Risk Assessment	"Risky" or "hazardous" drinking has been defined in the United States as more than 7 drinks per week or more than 3 drinks per occasion for women, and more than 14 drinks per week or more than 4 drinks per occasion for men. "Harmful drinking" describes persons who are currently experiencing physical, social, or psychological harm from alcohol use but do not meet criteria for dependence. Alcohol abuse and dependence are defined by specific criteria in the DSM-IV.
Screening Tests	The Alcohol Use Disorders Identification Test (AUDIT) is the most studied screening tool for detecting the full spectrum of alcohol-related problems in primary care settings. The 4-item CAGE is the most popular screening test for detecting alcohol abuse or dependence. TWEAK, a 5-item scale, and the T-ACE are designed to screen pregnant women for alcohol misuse. They detect lower levels of alcohol consumption that may pose risks during pregnancy. Clinicians may choose screening strategies that are appropriate for their clinical population and setting.
Timing of Screening	The optimal interval for screening and intervention is unknown. Patients with past alcohol problems, young adults, and other high-risk groups (e.g., smokers) may benefit most from frequent screening.
Interventions	Effective behavioral interventions to reduce risky/hazardous and harmful drinking include an initial counseling session of about 15 minutes, feedback, advice, and goal-setting. Most also include further assistance and followup. Resources that help clinicians deliver effective interventions include brief provider training or access to specially trained primary care practitioners or health educators, and the presence of office-level system supports (prompts, reminders, counseling algorithms, and patient education materials). All pregnant women and women contemplating pregnancy should be informed of the harmful effects of alcohol on the fetus. Referral or specialty treatment is recommended for individuals meeting the diagnostic criteria for alcohol dependence.
Balance of Benefits and Harms	Screening in primary care settings can accurately identify patients whose alcohol consumption does not meet criteria for alcohol dependence, but places them at risk for increased morbidity and mortality. Brief behavioral counseling interventions with followup produce small to moderate reductions in alcohol consumption that are sustained over 6 to 12 months or longer.	The evidence is insufficient to assess the potential benefits and harms of screening and behavioral counseling interventions in this population.
Other Relevant USPSTF Recommendations	The USPSTF has also made recommendations on screening for illicit drug use and counseling for tobacco cessation in adolescents, adults, and pregnant women. These recommendations are available at http://www.uspreventiveservicestaskforce.org/.

For a summary of the evidence systematically reviewed in making this recommendation, the full recommendation statement, and supporting documents, please go to http://www.uspreventiveservicestaskforce.org/.

ASPIRIN FOR THE PREVENTION OF CARDIOVASCULAR DISEASE

CLINICAL SUMMARY OF U.S. PREVENTIVE SERVICES TASK FORCE RECOMMENDATION

Population	Men age 45-79 years	Women age 55-79 years	Men age <45 years	Women age <55 years	Men & Women age ≥80 years
Recommendation	Encourage aspirin use when potential CVD benefit (MIs prevented) outweighs potential harm of GI hemorrhage.	Encourage aspirin use when potential CVD benefit (strokes prevented) outweighs potential harm of GI hemorrhage.	Do not encourage aspirin use for MI prevention.	Do not encourage aspirin use for stroke prevention.	No Recommendation
	Grade: A		Grade: D		Grade: I (Insufficient Evidence)
How to Use This Recommendation	Shared decisionmaking is strongly encouraged with individuals whose risk is close to (either above or below) the estimates of 10-year risk levels indicated below. As the potential CVD benefit increases above harms, the recommendation to take aspirin should become stronger. To determine whether the potential benefit of MIs prevented (men) and strokes prevented (women) outweighs the potential harm of increased GI hemorrhage, both 10-year CVD risk and age must be considered. **Risk level at which CVD events prevented (benefit) exceeds GI harms** **Men** 10-year CHD risk: Age 45-59 years ≥4%; Age 60-69 years ≥9%; Age 70-79 years ≥12%. **Women** 10-year stroke risk: Age 55-59 years ≥3%; Age 60-69 years ≥8%; Age 70-79 years ≥11%. **The table above applies to adults who are not taking NSAIDs and who do not have upper GI pain or a history of GI ulcers.** NSAID use and history of GI ulcers raise the risk of serious GI bleeding considerably and should be considered in determining the balance of benefits and harms. NSAID use combined with aspirin use approximately quadruples the risk of serious GI bleeding compared to the risk with aspirin use alone. The rate of serious bleeding in aspirin users is approximately 2-3 times higher in patients with a history of GI ulcers.				
Risk Assessment	**For men:** Risk factors for CHD include age, diabetes, total cholesterol level, HDL level, blood pressure, and smoking. CHD risk estimation tool: http://hp2010.nhlbihin.net/atpiii/calculator.asp **For women:** Risk factors for ischemic stroke include age, high blood pressure, diabetes, smoking, history of CVD, atrial fibrillation, and left ventricular hypertrophy. Stroke risk estimation tool: http://www.westernstroke.org/index.php?header_name=stroke_tools.gif&main=stroke_tools.php				
Other Relevant USPSTF Recommendations	The USPSTF has made recommendations on screening for abdominal aortic aneurysm, carotid artery stenosis, coronary heart disease, high blood pressure, lipid disorders, and peripheral arterial disease. These recommendations are available at http://www.uspreventiveservicestaskforce.org.				

Abbreviations: CHD = coronary heart disease. CVD = cardiovascular disease. GI = gastrointestinal. HDL = high-density lipoprotein. MI = myocardial infarction. NSAIDs = nonsteroidal anti-inflammatory drugs.

For a summary of the evidence systematically reviewed in making these recommendations, the full recommendation statement, and supporting documents, please go to http://www.uspreventiveservicestaskforce.org.

ROUTINE ASPIRIN OR NONSTEROIDAL ANTI-INFLAMMATORY DRUG (NSAID) USE FOR THE PRIMARY PREVENTION OF COLORECTAL CANCER

CLINICAL SUMMARY OF U.S. PREVENTIVE SERVICES TASK FORCE RECOMMENDATION

Population	Asymptomatic adults at average risk for colorectal cancer
Recommendation	Do not use aspirin or NSAIDs for the prevention of colorectal cancer. Grade: D

Risk Assessment	The major risk factors for colorectal cancer are older age (older than age 50 years), family history (having two or more first- or second-degree relatives with colorectal cancer), and African American race.
Balance of Benefits and Harms	Aspirin and NSAIDs, taken in higher doses for longer periods, reduce the incidence of adenomatous polyps. However, there is poor evidence that aspirin and NSAID use leads to a reduction in colorectal cancer-associated mortality. Aspirin increases the incidence of gastrointestinal bleeding and hemorrhagic stroke; NSAIDs increase the incidence of gastrointestinal bleeding and renal impairment, especially in the elderly. The USPSTF concluded that the harms outweigh the benefits of aspirin and NSAID use for the prevention of colorectal cancer.
Other Relevant USPSTF Recommendations	The USPSTF has made recommendations on screening for colorectal cancer and aspirin use for the prevention of cardiovascular disease. These recommendations are available at http://www.uspreventiveservicestaskforce.org/.

For a summary of the evidence systematically reviewed in making this recommendation, the full recommendation statement, and supporting documents, please go to http://www.uspreventiveservicestaskforce.org/.

SCREENING FOR BACTERIAL VAGINOSIS IN PREGNANCY TO PREVENT PRETERM DELIVERY

CLINICAL SUMMARY OF U.S. PREVENTIVE SERVICES TASK FORCE RECOMMENDATION

Population	Asymptomatic pregnant women without risk factors for preterm delivery	Asymptomatic pregnant women with risk factors for preterm delivery
Recommendation	Do not screen. **Grade: D**	No recommendation. **Grade: I (Insufficient Evidence)**
Risk Assessment	Risk factors of preterm delivery include: • African-American women. • Pelvic infection. • Previous preterm delivery. Bacterial vaginosis is more common among African-American women, women of low socioeconomic status, and women who have previously delivered low-birth-weight infants.	
Screening Tests	Bacterial vaginosis is diagnosed using Amsel's clinical criteria or Gram stain. When using Amsel's criteria, 3 out of 4 criteria must be met to make a clinical diagnosis: 1. Vaginal pH >4.7. 2. The presence of clue cells on wet mount. 3. Thin homogeneous discharge. 4. Amine 'fishy odor' when potassium hydroxide is added to the discharge.	
Screening Intervals	Not applicable.	
Treatment	Treatment is appropriate for pregnant women with symptomatic bacterial vaginosis infection. Oral metronidazole and oral clindamycin, as well as vaginal metronidazole gel or clindamycin cream, are used to treat bacterial vaginosis. The optimal treatment regimen is unclear.[1]	

[1]The Centers for Disease Control and Prevention (CDC) recommends 250 mg oral metronidazole 3 times a day for 7 days as the treatment for bacterial vaginosis in pregnancy.

For a summary of the evidence systematically reviewed in making these recommendations, the full recommendation statement, and supporting documents, please go to http://www.uspreventiveservicestaskforce.org.

SCREENING FOR ASYMPTOMATIC BACTERIURIA IN ADULTS

CLINICAL SUMMARY OF A U.S. PREVENTIVE SERVICES TASK FORCE RECOMMENDATION STATEMENT

Population	All pregnant women	Men and nonpregnant women
Recommendation	Screen with urine culture. Grade: A	Do not screen. Grade: D
Detection and Screening Tests	Asymptomatic bacteriuria can be reliably detected through urine culture. The presence of at least 105 colony-forming units per mL of urine, of a single uropathogen, and in a midstream clean-catch specimen is considered a positive test result.	
Screening Intervals	A clean-catch urine specimen should be collected for screening culture at 12-16 weeks' gestation or at the first prenatal visit, if later. The optimal frequency of subsequent urine testing during pregnancy is uncertain.	Do not screen.
Benefits of Detection and Early Treatment	The detection and treatment of asymptomatic bacteriuria with antibiotics significantly reduces the incidence of symptomatic maternal urinary tract infections and low birthweight.	Screening men and nonpregnant women for asymptomatic bacteriuria is ineffective in improving clinical outcomes.
Harms of Detection and Early Treatment	Potential harms associated with treatment of asymptomatic bacteriuria include: • Adverse effects from antibiotics. • Development of bacterial resistance.	
Other Relevant USPSTF Recommendations	Additional USPSTF recommendations involving screening for infectious conditions during pregnancy can be found at www.uspreventiveservicestaskforce.org/recommendations.htm#obstetric and www.uspreventiveservicestaskforce.org/recommendations.htm#infectious.	

For a summary of the evidence systematically reviewed in making these recommendations, the full recommendation statement, and supporting documents, please go to http://www.uspreventiveservicestaskforce.org.

SCREENING FOR BLADDER CANCER

CLINICAL SUMMARY OF U.S. PREVENTIVE SERVICES TASK FORCE RECOMMENDATION

Population	Asymptomatic adults
Recommendation	No recommendation. Grade: I (Insufficient Evidence)
Risk Assessment	Risk factors for bladder cancer include: • Smoking • Occupational exposure to carcinogens (e.g., rubber, chemical, and leather industries) • Male sex • Older age • White race • Infections caused by certain bladder parasites • Family or personal history of bladder cancer
Screening Tests	Screening tests for bladder cancer include: • Microscopic urinalysis for hematuria • Urine cytology • Urine biomarkers
Interventions	The principal treatment for superficial bladder cancer is transurethral resection of the bladder tumor, which may be combined with adjuvant radiation therapy, chemotherapy, biologic therapies, or photodynamic therapies. Radical cystectomy, often with adjuvant chemotherapy, is used in cases of surgically resectable invasive bladder cancer.
Balance of Benefits and Harms	There is inadequate evidence that treatment of screen-detected bladder cancer leads to improved morbidity or mortality. There is inadequate evidence on harms of screening for bladder cancer.
Suggestions for Practice	In deciding whether to screen for bladder cancer, clinicians should consider the following: • *Potential preventable burden:* early detection of tumors with malignant potential could have an important impact on the mortality rate of bladder cancer. • *Potential harms:* false-positive results may lead to anxiety and unneeded evaluations, diagnostic-related harms from cystoscopy and biopsy, harms from labeling and unnecessary treatments, and overdiagnosis. • *Current practice:* screening tests used in primary practice include microscopic urinalysis for hematuria and urine cytology; urine biomarkers are not commonly used in part because of cost. Patients with positive findings are typically referred to a urologist for further evaluation.
Other Relevant USPSTF Recommendations	Recommendations on screening for other types of cancer can be found at www.uspreventiveservicestaskforce.org.

For a summary of the evidence systematically reviewed in making these recommendations, the full recommendation statement, and supporting documents, please go to http://www.uspreventiveservicestaskforce.org.

GENETIC RISK ASSESSMENT AND BREAST CANCER SUSCEPTIBILITY GENE (*BRCA*) MUTATION TESTING FOR BREAST AND OVARIAN CANCER SUSCEPTIBILITY

CLINICAL SUMMARY OF U.S. PREVENTIVE SERVICES TASK FORCE RECOMMENDATION

Population	Women whose family history is not associated with an increased risk for deleterious mutations in the *BRCA1* or *BRCA2* gene	Women whose family history is associated with an increased risk for deleterious mutations in the *BRCA1* or *BRCA2* gene
Recommendation	Do not refer patients for genetic counseling or *BRCA* testing. Grade: D	Refer patients for genetic counseling and evaluation for *BRCA* testing. Grade: B
Risk Assessment	An increased-risk family history is defined as follows: For non-Ashkenazi Jewish women: 2 first-degree relatives with breast cancer, 1 of whom received the diagnosis at age 50 years or younger; a combination of 3 or more first- or second-degree relatives with breast cancer, regardless of age at diagnosis; a combination of both breast and ovarian cancer among first- and second-degree relatives; a first-degree relative with bilateral breast cancer; a combination of 2 or more first- or second-degree relatives with ovarian cancer, regardless of age at diagnosis; a first- or second-degree relative with both breast and ovarian cancer at any age; or a history of breast cancer in a male relative. For women of Ashkenazi Jewish heritage: an increased-risk family history includes any first-degree relative (or 2 second-degree relatives on the same side of the family) with breast or ovarian cancer. About 2% of adult women in the general population have an increased-risk family history as defined here. There are tools available to predict the risk for clinically important *BRCA* mutations, but these tools have not been verified in the general population. There is no evidence concerning the level of risk for a *BRCA* mutation that merits referral for genetic counseling.	
Screening Tests	Genetic counseling includes elements of counseling, risk assessment, pedigree analysis, and, in some cases, recommendations for testing for *BRCA* mutations in affected family members, the patient, or both. A *BRCA* test is typically ordered by a physician. When done together with genetic counseling, the test assures the linkage of testing with appropriate management decisions.	
Interventions	The interventions that can be offered to a woman with a deleterious *BRCA1* or *BRCA2* mutation or other increased risk for hereditary breast cancer include intensive screening, chemoprevention, prophylactic mastectomy or oophorectomy, or a combination.	
Balance of Benefits and Harms	Women without an increased-risk family history have a low risk for developing breast or ovarian cancer associated with *BRCA1* or *BRCA2* mutations. There are important adverse ethical, legal, and social consequences that can result from routine referral and testing of these women. Interventions such as prophylactic surgery, chemoprevention, or intensive screening have known harms. The potential harms of routine referral for genetic counseling or *BRCA* testing in these women outweigh the benefits.	Women with an increased-risk family history have an increased risk for developing breast or ovarian cancer associated with *BRCA1* or *BRCA2* mutations. The potential benefits of referral and discussion of testing and prophylactic treatment for these women may be substantial. The benefits of referring women with an increased-risk family history to suitably trained health care providers outweigh the harms.
Other Relevant USPSTF Recommendations	The USPSTF has made recommendations on mammography screening for breast cancer, screening for ovarian cancer, and chemoprevention of breast cancer. These recommendations are available at http://www.uspreventiveservicestaskforce.org/.	

For a summary of the evidence systematically reviewed in making this recommendation, the full recommendation statement, and supporting documents, please go to http://www.uspreventiveservicestaskforce.org/.

14

SCREENING FOR BREAST CANCER PART I: USING FILM MAMMOGRAPHY

CLINICAL SUMMARY OF 2009 U.S. PREVENTIVE SERVICES TASK FORCE RECOMMENDATION[1]

Population	Women aged 40-49 years	Women aged 50-74 years	Women aged ≥75 years
Recommendation	Individualize decision to begin biennial screening according to the patient's circumstances and values. Grade: C	Screen every 2 years. Grade: B	No recommendation. Grade: I (Insufficient Evidence)
Risk Assessment	This recommendation applies to women aged ≥40 years who are not at increased risk by virtue of a known genetic mutation or history of chest radiation. Increasing age is the most important risk factor for most women.		
Screening Tests	Standardization of film mammography has led to improved quality. Refer patients to facilities certified under the Mammography Quality Standards Act (MQSA), listed at http://www.accessdata.fda.gov/scripts/cdrh/cfdocs/cfMQSA/mqsa.cfm		
Timing of Screening	Evidence indicates that biennial screening is optimal. A biennial schedule preserves most of the benefit of annual screening and cuts the harms nearly in half. A longer interval may reduce the benefit.		
Balance of Benefits and Harms	There is convincing evidence that screening with film mammography reduces breast cancer mortality, with a greater absolute reduction for women aged 50 to 74 years than for younger women. Harms of screening include psychological harms, additional medical visits, imaging, and biopsies in women without cancer, inconvenience due to false-positive screening results, harms of unnecessary treatment, and radiation exposure. Harms seem moderate for each age group. False-positive results are a greater concern for younger women; treatment of cancer that would not become clinically apparent during a woman's life (overdiagnosis) is an increasing problem as women age.		
Rationale for No Recommendation (I Statement)			Among women 75 years or older, evidence of benefit is lacking.
Other Relevant USPSTF Recommendations	USPSTF recommendations on screening for genetic susceptibility for breast cancer and chemoprevention of breast cancer are available at http://www.uspreventiveservicestaskforce.org.		

[1] The U.S. Department of Health and Human Services, in implementing the Affordable Care Act under the standard it sets out in revised Section 2713(a)(5) of the Public Health Service Act, utilizes the 2002 recommendation on breast cancer screening of the U.S. Preventive Services Task Force. For clinical summary of 2002 Recommendation, see Appendix F.

For a summary of the evidence systematically reviewed in making these recommendations, the full recommendation statement, and supporting documents, please go to http://www.uspreventiveservicestaskforce.org.

SCREENING FOR BREAST CANCER PART II: USING METHODS OTHER THAN FILM MAMMOGRAPHY

CLINICAL SUMMARY OF 2009 U.S. PREVENTIVE SERVICES TASK FORCE RECOMMENDATION[1]

Population	Women aged ≥40 years			
Screening Method	Digital mammography	Magnetic resonance imaging (MRI)	Clinical breast examination (CBE)	Breast self-examination (BSE)
Recommendation	Grade: I (Insufficient Evidence)			Grade: D
Rationale for No Recommendation or Negative Recommendation	Evidence is lacking for benefits of digital mammography and MRI of the breast as substitutes for film mammography.		Evidence of CBE's additional benefit, beyond mammography, is inadequate.	Adequate evidence suggests that BSE does not reduce breast cancer mortality.
Considerations for Practice				
Potential Preventable Burden	For younger women and women with dense breast tissue, overall detection is somewhat better with digital mammography.	Contrast-enhanced MRI has been shown to detect more cases of cancer in very high-risk populations than does mammography.	Indirect evidence suggests that when CBE is the only test available, it may detect a significant proportion of cancer cases.	
Potential Harms	It is not certain whether overdiagnosis occurs more often with digital than with film mammography.	Contrast-enhanced MRI requires injection of contrast material. MRI yields many more false-positive results and potentially more overdiagnosis than mammography.	Harms of CBE include false-positive results, which lead to anxiety, unnecessary visits, imaging, and biopsies.	Harms of BSE include the same potential harms as for CBE and may be larger in magnitude.
Costs	Digital mammography is more expensive than film.	MRI is much more expensive than mammography.	Costs of CBE are primarily opportunity costs to clinicians.	Costs of BSE are primarily opportunity costs to clinicians.
Current Practice	Some clinical practices are now switching to digital equipment.	MRI is not currently used to screen women of average risk.	No standard approach or reporting standards are in place.	The number of clinicians who teach BSE to patients is unknown; it is likely that few clinicians teach BSE to all women.

[1] The U.S. Department of Health and Human Services, in implementing the Affordable Care Act under the standard it sets out in revised Section 2713(a)(5) of the Public Health Service Act, utilizes the 2002 recommendation on breast cancer screening of the U.S. Preventive Services Task Force. For clinical summary of 2002 Recommendation, see Appendix F.

For a summary of the evidence systematically reviewed in making these recommendations, the full recommendation statement, and supporting documents, please go to http://www.uspreventiveservicestaskforce.org.

PRIMARY CARE INTERVENTIONS TO PROMOTE BREASTFEEDING

CLINICAL SUMMARY OF U.S. PREVENTIVE SERVICES TASK FORCE RECOMMENDATION

Population	Pregnant women	New mothers	The mother's partner, other family members, and friends	Infants and young children
Recommendation	Promote and support breastfeeding. Grade: B			

Benefits of Breastfeeding	Mothers Less likelihood of breast and ovarian cancer		Infants Fewer ear infections, lower-respiratory-tract infections, and gastrointestinal infections	Young children Less likelihood of asthma, type 2 diabetes, and obesity
Interventions to Promote Breastfeeding	Interventions to promote and support breastfeeding have been found to increase the rates of initiation, duration, and exclusivity of breastfeeding. Consider multiple strategies, including: • Formal breastfeeding education for mothers and families • Direct support of mothers during breastfeeding • Training of primary care staff about breastfeeding and techniques for breastfeeding support • Peer support Interventions that include both prenatal and postnatal components may be most effective at increasing breastfeeding duration. In rare circumstances, for example for mothers with HIV and infants with galactosemia, breastfeeding is not recommended. Interventions to promote breastfeeding should empower individuals to make informed choices supported by the best available evidence.			
Implementation	System-level interventions with senior leadership support may be more likely to be sustained over time.			

For a summary of the evidence systematically reviewed in making these recommendations, the full recommendation statement, and supporting documents, please go to http://www.uspreventiveservicestaskforce.org.

SCREENING FOR CAROTID ARTERY STENOSIS

CLINICAL SUMMARY OF U.S. PREVENTIVE SERVICES TASK FORCE RECOMMENDATION

Population	Adult general population[1]
Recommendation	Do not screen with ultrasound or other screening tests. Grade: D

Risk Assessment	The major risk factors for carotid artery stenosis (CAS) include: older age, male gender, hypertension, smoking, hypercholesterolemia, and heart disease. However, accurate, reliable risk assessment tools are not available.
Balance of Benefits and Harms	Harms outweigh benefits. In the general population, screening with carotid duplex ultrasound would result in more false-positive results than true positive results. This would lead either to surgeries that are not indicated or to confirmatory angiography. As the result of these procedures, some people would suffer serious harms (death, stroke, and myocardial infarction) that outweigh the potential benefit surgical treatment may have in preventing stroke.
Other Relevant Recommendations from the USPSTF	Adults should be screened for hypertension, hyperlipidemia, and smoking. Clinicians should discuss aspirin chemoprevention with patients at increased risk for cardiovascular disease. These recommendations and related evidence are available at http://www.uspreventiveservicestaskforce.org.

[1]This recommendation applies to adults without neurological symptoms and without a history of transient ischemic attacks (TIA) or stroke. If otherwise eligible, an individual who has a carotid area TIA should be evaluated promptly for consideration of carotid endarterectomy.

For a summary of the evidence systematically reviewed in making these recommendations, the full recommendation statement, and supporting documents, please go to http://www.uspreventiveservicestaskforce.org.

SCREENING FOR CERVICAL CANCER

CLINICAL SUMMARY OF U.S. PREVENTIVE SERVICES TASK FORCE RECOMMENDATION

Population	Women ages 21 to 65	Women ages 30 to 65	Women younger than age 21	Women older than age 65 who have had adequate prior screening and are not high risk	Women after hysterectomy with removal of the cervix and with no history of high-grade precancer or cervical cancer	Women younger than age 30
Recommendation	Screen with cytology (Pap smear) every 3 years. Grade: A	Screen with cytology every 3 years or co-testing (cytology/HPV testing) every 5 years Grade: A	Do not screen. Grade: D	Do not screen. Grade: D	Do not screen. Grade: D	Do not screen with HPV testing (alone or with cytology) Grade: D

Risk Assessment	Human papillomavirus (HPV) infection is associated with nearly all cases of cervical cancer. Other factors that put a woman at increased risk of cervical cancer include HIV infection, a compromised immune system, in utero exposure to diethylstilbestrol, and previous treatment of a high-grade precancerous lesion or cervical cancer.
Screening Tests and Interval	Screening women ages 21 to 65 years every 3 years with cytology provides a reasonable balance between benefits and harms. Screening with cytology more often than every 3 years confers little additional benefit, with large increases in harms. HPV testing combined with cytology (co-testing) every 5 years in women ages 30 to 65 years offers a comparable balance of benefits and harms, and is therefore a reasonable alternative for women in this age group who would prefer to extend the screening interval.
Timing of Screening	Screening earlier than age 21 years, regardless of sexual history, leads to more harms than benefits. Clinicians and patients should base the decision to end screening on whether the patient meets the criteria for adequate prior testing and appropriate follow-up, per established guidelines.
Interventions	Screening aims to identify high-grade precancerous cervical lesions to prevent development of cervical cancer and early-stage asymptomatic invasive cervical cancer. High-grade lesions may be treated with ablative and excisional therapies, including cryotherapy, laser ablation, loop excision, and cold knife conization. Early-stage cervical cancer may be treated with surgery (hysterectomy) or chemoradiation.
Balance of Benefits and Harms	The benefits of screening with cytology every 3 years substantially outweigh the harms.	The benefits of screening with co-testing (cytology/HPV testing) every 5 years outweigh the harms.	The harms of screening earlier than age 21 years outweigh the benefits.	The benefits of screening after age 65 years do not outweigh the potential harms.	The harms of screening after hysterectomy outweigh the benefits.	The potential harms of screening with HPV testing (alone or with cytology) outweigh the potential benefits.
Other Relevant USPSTF Recommendations	The USPSTF has made recommendations on screening for breast cancer and ovarian cancer, as well as genetic risk assessment and *BRCA* mutation testing for breast and ovarian cancer susceptibility. These recommendations are available at http://www.uspreventiveservicestaskforce.org/.

For a summary of the evidence systematically reviewed in making this recommendation, the full recommendation statement, and supporting documents, please go to http://www.uspreventiveservicestaskforce.org/.

SCREENING FOR CHLAMYDIAL INFECTION

CLINICAL SUMMARY OF U.S. PREVENTIVE SERVICES TASK FORCE RECOMMENDATION

Population	Non-pregnant women			Pregnant women			Men
	24 years and younger	25 years and older		24 years and younger	25 years and older		
	Includes adolescents	Not at increased risk	At increased risk	Includes adolescents	Not at increased risk	At increased risk	
Recommendation	Screen if sexually active. Grade: A	Do not automatically screen. Grade: C	Screen. Grade: A	Screen. Grade: B	Do not automatically screen. Grade: C	Screen. Grade: B	No recommendation. Grade: I (Insufficient Evidence[1])

Risk Assessment	**Age:** Women and men aged 24 years and younger are at greatest risk. **History of:** previous Chlamydial infection or other sexually transmitted infections, new or multiple sexual partners, inconsistent condom use, sex work. **Demographics:** African-Americans and Hispanic women and men have higher prevalence rates than the general population in many communities.
Screening Tests	Nucleic acid amplification tests (NAATs) can identify chlamydial infection in asymptomatic women (non-pregnant and pregnant) and asymptomatic men. NAATs have high specificity and sensitivity and can be used with urine and vaginal swabs.
Screening Intervals	**Non-Pregnant Women** The optimal interval for screening is not known. The CDC recommends that women at increased risk be screened at least annually.[2] **Pregnant Women** For women 24 years and younger and older women at increased risk: Screen at the first prenatal visit. For patients at continuing risk, or who are newly at risk: Screen in the 3rd trimester. / Not applicable
Treatment	The Centers for Disease Control and Prevention has outlined appropriate treatment at: http://www.cdc.gov/STD/treatment. Test and/or treat partners of patients treated for Chlamydial infection.

[1] Chlamydial infection results in few sequelae in men. Therefore, the major benefit of screening men would be to reduce the likelihood that infected and untreated men would pass the infection to sexual partners. There is no evidence that screening men reduces the long-term consequences of chlamydial infection in women. Because of this lack of evidence, the USPSTF was not able to assess the balance of benefits and harms, and concluded that the evidence is insufficient to recommend for or against routinely screening men.

[2] Centers for Disease Control and Prevention. Sexually transmitted diseases treatment guidelines. 2006. *MMWR* 2006. 55(No. RR-11).

For a summary of the evidence systematically reviewed in making these recommendations, the full recommendation statement, and supporting documents, please go to http://www.uspreventiveservicestaskforce.org.

SCREENING FOR CHRONIC OBSTRUCTIVE PULMONARY DISEASE USING SPIROMETRY

CLINICAL SUMMARY OF U.S. PREVENTIVE SERVICES TASK FORCE RECOMMENDATION

Population	Adult general population
Recommendation	Do not screen for chronic obstructive pulmonary disease using spirometry. Grade: D

Additional Population Information	This screening recommendation applies to healthy adults who do not recognize or report respiratory symptoms to a clinician. It does not apply to individuals with a family history of alpha-1 antitrypsin deficiency.
Risk Assessment	Risk factors for COPD include: • Current or past tobacco use. • Exposure to occupational and environmental pollutants. • Age 40 or older.
Screening Tests[1]	Spirometry can be performed in a primary care physician's office or a pulmonary testing laboratory. The USPSTF did not review evidence comparing the accuracy of spirometry performed in primary care versus referral settings. For individuals who present to clinicians complaining of chronic cough, increased sputum production, wheezing, or dyspnea, spirometry would be indicated as a diagnostic test for COPD, asthma, and other pulmonary diseases.
Other Approaches to the Prevention of Pulmonary Illnesses	These services should be offered to patients regardless of COPD status: • All current smokers should receive smoking cessation counseling and be offered pharmacologic therapies demonstrated to increase cessation rates. • All patients 50 years of age or older should be offered influenza immunization annually. • All patients 65 years of age or older should be offered one-time pneumococcal immunization.
Other Relevant USPSTF Recommendations	Clinicians should screen all adults for tobacco use and provide tobacco cessation interventions for those who use tobacco products. The USPSTF tobacco cessation counseling recommendation and supporting evidence are available at http://www.uspreventiveservicestaskforce.org/uspstf/uspstbac.htm.

[1]The potential benefit of spirometry-based screening for COPD is prevention of one or more exacerbations by treating patients found to have an airflow obstruction previously undetected. However, even in groups with the greatest prevalence of airflow obstruction, hundreds of patients would need to be screened with spirometry to defer one exacerbation.

For a summary of the evidence systematically reviewed in making these recommendations, the full recommendation statement, and supporting documents, please go to http://www.uspreventiveservicestaskforce.org.

SCREENING FOR COLORECTAL CANCER

CLINICAL SUMMARY OF U.S. PREVENTIVE SERVICES TASK FORCE RECOMMENDATION

Population	Adults age 50 to 75[1] years	Adults age 76 to 85 years[1]	Adults older than 85 years[1]
Recommendation	Screen with high sensitivity fecal occult blood testing (FOBT), sigmoidoscopy, or colonoscopy. Grade: A	Do not automatically screen. Grade: C	Do not screen. Grade: D
	For all populations, evidence is insufficient to assess the benefits and harms of screening with computerized tomography colonography (CTC) and fecal DNA testing. Grade: I (Insufficient Evidence)		

Screening Tests	High sensitivity FOBT, sigmoidoscopy with FOBT, and colonoscopy are effective in decreasing colorectal cancer mortality. The risks and benefits of these screening methods vary. Colonoscopy and flexible sigmoidoscopy (to a lesser degree) entail possible serious complications.
Screening Test Intervals	Intervals for recommended screening strategies: • Annual screening with high-sensitivity fecal occult blood testing • Sigmoidoscopy every 5 years, with high-sensitivity fecal occult blood testing every 3 years • Screening colonoscopy every 10 years
Balance of Benefits and Harms	The benefits of screening outweigh the potential harms for 50- to 75-year-olds.	The likelihood that detection and early intervention will yield a mortality benefit declines after age 75 because of the long average time between adenoma development and cancer diagnosis.
Implementation	Focus on strategies that maximize the number of individuals who get screened. Practice shared decisionmaking; discussions with patients should incorporate information on test quality and availability. Individuals with a personal history of cancer or adenomatous polyps are followed by a surveillance regimen, and screening guidelines are not applicable.
Other Relevant USPSTF Recommendations	The USPSTF recommends against the use of aspirin or nonsteroidal anti-inflammatory drugs for the primary prevention of colorectal cancer. This recommendation is available at http://www.uspreventiveservicestaskforce.org.

[1]These recommendations do not apply to individuals with specific inherited syndromes (Lynch Syndrome or Familial Adenomatous Polyposis) or those with inflammatory bowel disease.

For a summary of the evidence systematically reviewed in making these recommendations, the full recommendation statement, and supporting documents, please go to http://www.uspreventiveservicestaskforce.org.

USING NONTRADITIONAL RISK FACTORS IN CORONARY HEART DISEASE RISK ASSESSMENT

CLINICAL SUMMARY OF U.S. PREVENTIVE SERVICES TASK FORCE RECOMMENDATION

Population	Asymptomatic men and women with no history of coronary heart disease (CHD), diabetes, or any CHD risk equivalent
Recommendation	No recommendation. Grade: I (Insufficient Evidence)
Risk Assessment	This recommendation applies to adult men and women classified at intermediate 10-year risk for CHD (10% to 20%) by traditional risk factors.
Importance	Coronary heart disease (CHD) is the most common cause of death in adults in the United States. Treatment to prevent CHD events by modifying risk factors is currently based on the Framingham risk model. If the classification of individuals at intermediate risk could be improved by using additional risk factors, treatment to prevent CHD might be targeted more effectively. Risk factors not currently part of the Framingham model (nontraditional risk factors) include high sensitivity C-reactive protein (hs-CRP), ankle-brachial index (ABI), leukocyte count, fasting blood glucose level, periodontal disease, carotid intima-media thickness, electron beam computed tomography, homocysteine level, and lipoprotein(a) level.
Balacne of Benefits and Harms	There is insufficient evidence to determine the percentage of intermediate-risk individuals who would be reclassified by screening with nontraditional risk factors, other than hs-CRP and ABI. For individuals reclassified as high-risk on the basis of hs-CRP or ABI scores, data are not available to determine whether they benefit from additional treatments. Little evidence is available to determine the harms of using nontraditional risk factors in screening. Potential harms include lifelong use of medications without proven benefit and psychological and other harms from being misclassified in a higher risk category.
Suggestions for practice	Clinicians should continue to use the Framingham model to assess CHD risk and guide risk-based preventive therapy. Adding nontraditional risk factors to CHD assessment would require additional patient and clinical staff time and effort. Routinely screening with nontraditional risk factors could result in lost opportunities to provide other important health services of proven benefit.
Other Relevant USPSTF Recommendations	USPSTF recommendations on risk assessment for CHD, the use of aspirin to prevent cardiovascular disease, and screening for high blood pressure can be accessed at http://www.uspreventiveservicestaskforce.org.

For a summary of the evidence systematically reviewed in making these recommendations, the full recommendation statement, and supporting documents, please go to http://www.uspreventiveservicestaskforce.org.

SCREENING FOR DEPRESSION IN ADULTS

CLINICAL SUMMARY OF U.S. PREVENTIVE SERVICES TASK FORCE RECOMMENDATION

Population	Nonpregnant adults 18 years or older	
Recommendation	Screen when staff-assisted depression care supports[1] are in place to assure accurate diagnosis, effective treatment, and followup. Grade: B	Do not automatically screen when staff-assisted depression care supports[1] are not in place. Grade: C
Risk Assessment	Persons at increased risk for depression are considered at risk throughout their lifetime. Groups at increased risk include persons with other psychiatric disorders, including substance misuse; persons with a family history of depression; persons with chronic medical diseases; and persons who are unemployed or of lower socioeconomic status. Also, women are at increased risk compared with men. However, the presence of risk factors alone cannot distinguish depressed patients from nondepressed patients.	
Screening Tests	Simple screening questions may perform as well as more complex instruments. Any positive screening test result should trigger a full diagnostic interview using standard diagnostic criteria.	
Timing of Screening	The optimal interval for screening is unknown. In older adults, significant depressive symptoms are associated with common life events, including medical illness, cognitive decline, bereavement, and institutional placement in residential or inpatient settings.	
Balance of Benefits and Harms	Limited evidence suggests that screening for depression in the absence of staff-assisted depression care does not improve depression outcomes.	
Suggestions for Practice	"Staff-assisted depression care supports" refers to clinical staff that assists the primary care clinician by providing some direct depression care and/or coordination, case management, or mental health treatment.	
Relevant USPSTF Recommendations	Related USPSTF recommendations on screening for suicidality and screening children and adolescents for depression are available at http://www.uspreventiveservicestaskforce.org.	

[1]Go to the Suggestions for Practice section of this figure for further explanation.

For a summary of the evidence systematically reviewed in making these recommendations, the full recommendation statement, and supporting documents, please go to http://www.uspreventiveservicestaskforce.org.

SCREENING FOR TYPE 2 DIABETES MELLITUS IN ADULTS

CLINICAL SUMMARY OF U.S. PREVENTIVE SERVICES TASK FORCE RECOMMENDATION

Population	Asymptomatic adults with sustained blood pressure greater than 135/80 mm Hg	Asymptomatic adults with sustained blood pressure 135/80 mm Hg or lower
Recommendation	Screen for type 2 diabetes mellitus. Grade: B	No recommendation. Grade: I (Insufficient Evidence)
Risk Assessment	These recommendations apply to adults with no symptoms of type 2 diabetes mellitus or evidence of possible complications of diabetes. Blood pressure measurement is an important predictor of cardiovascular complications in people with type 2 diabetes mellitus. The first step in applying this recommendation should be measurement of blood pressure (BP). Adults with treated or untreated BP >135/80 mm Hg should be screened for diabetes.	
Screening Tests	Three tests have been used to screen for diabetes: • Fasting plasma glucose (FPG). • 2-hour postload plasma. • Hemoglobin A1c. The American Diabetes Association (ADA) recommends screening with FPG, defines diabetes as FPG ≥ 126 mg/dL, and recommends confirmation with a repeated screening test on a separate day.	
Screening Intervals	The optimal screening interval is not known. The ADA, on the basis of expert opinion, recommends an interval of every 3 years.	
Suggestions for practice regarding insufficient evidence	When BP is ≤ 135/80 mm Hg, screening may be considered on an individual basis when knowledge of diabetes status would help inform decisions about coronary heart disease (CHD) preventive strategies, including consideration of lipid-lowering agents or aspirin. To determine whether screening would be helpful on an individual basis, information about 10-year CHD risk must be considered. For example, if CHD risk without diabetes was 17% and risk with diabetes was >20%, screening for diabetes would be helpful because diabetes status would determine lipid treatment. In contrast, if risk without diabetes was 10% and risk with diabetes was 15%, screening would not affect the decision to use lipid-lowering treatment.	
Other relevant information from the USPSTF and the Community Preventive Services Task Force	Evidence and USPSTF recommendations regarding blood pressure, diet, physical activity, and obesity are available at http://www.uspreventiveservicestaskforce.org. The reviews and recommendations of the Community Preventive Services Task Force may be found at http://www.thecommunityguide.org.	

For a summary of the evidence systematically reviewed in making these recommendations, the full recommendation statement, and supporting documents, please go to http://www.uspreventiveservicestaskforce.org.

25

FOLIC ACID FOR THE PREVENTION OF NEURAL TUBE DEFECTS

CLINICAL SUMMARY OF U.S. PREVENTIVE SERVICES TASK FORCE RECOMMENDATION

Population	Women planning a pregnancy or capable of becoming pregnant
Recommendation	Take a daily vitamin supplement containing 0.4 to 0.8 mg (400 to 800 μg) of folic acid. Grade: A
Risk Assessment	Risk factors include: • A personal or family history of a pregnancy affected by a neural tube defect • The use of certain antiseizure medications • Mutations in folate-related enzymes • Maternal diabetes • Maternal obesity **Note:** This recommendation does not apply to women who have had a previous pregnancy affected by neural tube defects or women taking certain antiseizure medicines. These women may be advised to take higher doses of folic acid.
Timing of Medication	Start supplementation at least 1 month before conception. Continue through first 2 to 3 months of pregnancy.
Recommendations of Others	ACOG, AAFP, and most other organizations recommend 4 mg/d for women with a history of a pregnancy affected by a neural tube defect.

Abbreviations: AAFP = American Academy of Family Physicians; ACOG = American College of Obstetricians and Gynecologists.

For a summary of the evidence systematically reviewed in making these recommendations, the full recommendation statement, and supporting documents, please go to http://www.uspreventiveservicestaskforce.org.

SCREENING FOR GENITAL HERPES

CLINICAL SUMMARY OF U.S. PREVENTIVE SERVICES TASK FORCE RECOMMENDATION

Population	Asymptomatic pregnant women	Asymptomatic adolescents and adults
Recommendation	Do not screen for herpes simplex virus. Grade: D	Do not screen for herpes simplex virus. Grade: D
Screening Tests	Methods for detecting herpes simplex virus include viral culture, polymerase chain reaction, and antibody-based tests, such as the western blot assay and type-specific glycoprotein G serological tests.	
Interventions	There is limited evidence that the use of antiviral therapy in women with a history of recurrent infection, or performance of cesarean delivery in women with active herpes lesions at the time of delivery, decreases neonatal herpes infection. There is also limited evidence of the safety of antiviral therapy in pregnant women and neonates.	Antiviral therapy improves health outcomes in symptomatic persons (e.g., those with multiple recurrences); however, there is no evidence that the use of antiviral therapy improves health outcomes in those with asymptomatic infection. There are multiple efficacious regimens that may be used to prevent the recurrence of clinical genital herpes.
Balance of Benefits and Harms	The potential harms of screening asymptomatic pregnant women include false-positive test results, labeling, and anxiety, as well as false-negative tests and false reassurance, although these potential harms are not well studied. The USPSTF determined that there are no benefits associated with screening, and therefore the potential harms outweigh the benefits.	The potential harms of screening asymptomatic adolescents and adults include false-positive test results, labeling, and anxiety, although these potential harms are not well studied. The USPSTF determined the benefits of screening are minimal, at best, and the potential harms outweigh the potential benefits.
Other Relevant USPSTF Recommendations	The USPSTF has made recommendations on screening for chlamydia, gonorrhea, HIV, and several other sexually transmitted infections. These recommendations are available at http://www.uspreventiveservicestaskforce.org/.	

For a summary of the evidence systematically reviewed in making this recommendation, the full recommendation statement, and supporting documents, please go to http://www.uspreventiveservicestaskforce.org/.

SCREENING FOR GESTATIONAL DIABETES MELLITUS

CLINICAL SUMMARY OF U.S. PREVENTIVE SERVICES TASK FORCE RECOMMENDATION

Population	Pregnant women who have not previously been diagnosed with diabetes
Recommendation	No recommendation. Grade: I (Insufficient Evidence[1]).
Risk Assessment	Women at increased risk of developing gestational diabetes mellitus (GDM) include those who: • Are obese. • Are older than 25 years. • Have a family history of diabetes. • Have a history of GDM. • Are of certain ethnic groups (Hispanic, American Indian, Asian, or African-American).
Balacne of Benefits and Harms	The current evidence is insufficient to assess the balance between the benefits and harms of screening women for GDM either before or after 24 weeks gestation. Harms of screening include short-term anxiety in some women with positive screening results, and inconvenience to many women and medical practices because most positive screening tests are likely false-positives.
Suggestions for Practice	Until there is better evidence, clinicians should discuss screening for GDM with their patients and make case-by-case decisions. The discussion should include information about the uncertain benefits and harms as well as the frequency and uncertain meaning of a positive screening test result. If a decision is made to screen for GDM:
Screening Tests	The screening test most commonly used in the United States is an initial 50-gram 1-hour glucose challenge test (GCT). If the result on the GCT is abnormal, the patient undergoes a 100-gram 3-hour oral glucose tolerance test (OGTT). Two or more abnormal values on the OGTT are considered a diagnosis of GDM.
Screening Intervals	Most screening is conducted between 24 and 28 weeks gestation. There is little evidence about the value of earlier screening.
Other Approaches to Prevention	Nearly all pregnant women should be encouraged to: • Achieve moderate weight gain based on their pre-pregnancy body mass index. • Participate in physical activity.

[1]The current evidence is insufficient to establish the balance of benefits and harms for screening for gestational diabetes mellitus, either before or after 24 weeks gestation.

For a summary of the evidence systematically reviewed in making these recommendations, the full recommendation statement, and supporting documents, please go to http://www.uspreventiveservicestaskforce.org.

SCREENING FOR GLAUCOMA

CLINICAL SUMMARY OF U.S. PREVENTIVE SERVICES TASK FORCE RECOMMENDATION

Population	Asymptomatic adults
Recommendation	No recommendation. Grade: I (Insufficient Evidence)

Risk Assessment	The primary risk factor for developing primary open-angle glaucoma (POAG) is increased intraocular pressure. Other important risk factors are family history, older age, and being of African American descent. Additional risk factors may include decreased central cornea thickness, low diastolic perfusion pressure, diabetes, and severe myopia.
Screening Tests	The diagnosis of POAG is not made on the basis of a single test, but on the finding of characteristic degenerative changes in the optic disc, along with a loss of visual field sensitivity. Perimetry assesses visual field loss by mapping a patient's response to visual stimuli presented in various locations within the visual field. Perimetry may be performed by manual or automated methods. Several consistent perimetry measurements are needed to establish the presence of defects. Dilated opthalmoscopy or slit lamp examinations are used by specialists to examine changes in the optic disc; however, there is wide variability in its reliability for detecting glaucomatous optic disc progression.
Interventions	The primary treatments for POAG reduce intraocular pressure; these include medications, laser therapy, or surgery. These treatments can effectively reduce the development and progression of small visual field defects. However, their effectiveness in reducing impairment in vision-related function is uncertain. Harms caused by these interventions include formation of cataracts, harms resulting from cataract surgery, and harms of topical medication.
Balance of Benefits and Harms	Because of the uncertainty of the magnitude of benefit from early treatment and given the known harms of screening and early treatment, the USPSTF could not determine the balance between the benefits and harms of screening for glaucoma.
Other Relevant USPSTF Recommendations	The USPSTF has also made a recommendation on screening for impaired visual acuity in older adults. This recommendation is available at http://www.uspreventiveservicestaskforce.org/.

For a summary of the evidence systematically reviewed in making this recommendation, the full recommendation statement, and supporting documents, please go to http://www.uspreventiveservicestaskforce.org/.

29

SCREENING FOR GONORRHEA

CLINICAL SUMMARY OF U.S. PREVENTIVE SERVICES TASK FORCE RECOMMENDATION

Population	Sexually active women, including those who are pregnant, who are at increased risk for infection	Men who are at increased risk for infection	Men and women who are at low risk for infection	Pregnant women who are not at increased risk for infection
Recommendation	Screen for gonorrhea. Grade: B	No recommendation. Grade: I (Insufficient Evidence)	Do not screen for gonorrhea. Grade: D	No recommendation. Grade: I (Insufficient Evidence)

Risk Assessment	Women and men younger than age 25 years—including sexually active adolescents—are at highest risk for gonorrhea infection. Risk factors for gonorrhea include a history of previous gonorrhea infection, other sexually transmitted infections, new or multiple sexual partners, inconsistent condom use, sex work, and drug use. Risk factors for pregnant women are the same as for non-pregnant women.
Screening Tests	Vaginal culture is an accurate screening test when transport conditions are suitable. Newer screening tests, including nucleic acid amplification and hybridization tests, have demonstrated improved sensitivity and comparable specificity when compared with cervical culture. Some newer tests can be used with urine and vaginal swabs, which enables screening when a pelvic examination is not performed.
Timing of Screening	Screening is recommended at the first prenatal visit for pregnant women who are in a high-risk group for gonorrhea infection. For pregnant women who are at continued risk, and for those who acquire a new risk factor, a second screening should be conducted during the third trimester. The optimal interval for screening in the non-pregnant population is not known.
Interventions	Genital gonorrhea infection in men and women, including pregnant women, may be treated with a third-generation cephalosporin. Because of increased prevalence of resistant organisms, fluoroquinolones should not be used to treat gonorrhea. Current guidelines for treating gonorrhea infection are available from the Centers for Disease Control and Prevention (http://www.cdc.gov/std/treatment).
Balance of Benefits and Harms	The USPSTF concluded that the benefits of screening women at increased risk for gonorrhea infection outweigh the potential harms. / The USPSTF could not determine the balance of benefits and harms of screening for gonorrhea in men at increased risk for infection. / Given the low prevalence of gonorrhea infection in the general population, the USPSTF concluded that the potential harms of screening in low-prevalence populations outweigh the benefits. / The USPSTF could not determine the balance between the benefits and harms of screening for gonorrhea in pregnant women who are not at increased risk for infection.
Other Relevant USPSTF Recommendations	The USPSTF has also made a recommendation on ocular prophylaxis in newborns for gonococcal ophthalmia neonatorum. This recommendation is available at http://www.uspreventiveservicestaskforce.org/.

For a summary of the evidence systematically reviewed in making this recommendation, the full recommendation statement, and supporting documents, please go to http://www.uspreventiveservicestaskforce.org/.

SCREENING FOR HEMOCHROMATOSIS

CLINICAL SUMMARY OF U.S. PREVENTIVE SERVICES TASK FORCE RECOMMENDATION

Population	Asymptomatic general population
Recommendation	Do not screen for hereditary hemochromatosis. Grade: D

Risk Assessment	Clinically recognized hereditary hemochromatosis is primarily associated with mutations on the hemochromatosis (*HFE*) gene. Although this is a relatively common mutation in the U.S. population, only a small subset will develop symptoms of hemochromatosis. An even smaller proportion of these individuals will develop advanced stages of clinical disease.
Screening Tests	Genetic screening for *HFE* mutations can accurately identify individuals at risk for hereditary hemochromatosis. However, identifying an individual with the genotypic predisposition does not accurately predict the future risk for disease manifestation.
Interventions	Therapeutic phlebotomy is the main treatment for hereditary hemochromatosis. Phlebotomy is generally thought to have few side effects.
Balance of Benefits and Harms	• Screening could lead to identification of a large number of individuals who possess the high-risk genotype but may never manifest the clinical disease. This may result in unnecessary surveillance and diagnostic procedures, labeling, anxiety, and, potentially, unnecessary treatments. • There is poor evidence that early therapeutic phlebotomy improves morbidity and mortality in individuals with screening-detected versus clinically-detected hemochromatosis. • The USPSTF concluded that the potential harms of genetic screening for hereditary hemochromatosis outweigh the potential benefits.
Other Relevant USPSTF Recommendations	The USPSTF has also made recommendations on genetic testing for mutations in the breast cancer susceptibility gene to predict breast and ovarian cancer susceptibility. These recommendations are available at http://www.uspreventiveservicestaskforce.org/.

For a summary of the evidence systematically reviewed in making this recommendation, the full recommendation statement, and supporting documents, please go to http://www.uspreventiveservicestaskforce.org/.

SCREENING FOR HEPATITIS B VIRUS INFECTION

CLINICAL SUMMARY OF U.S. PREVENTIVE SERVICES TASK FORCE RECOMMENDATION

Population	General asymptomatic population
Recommendation	Do not screen for hepatitis B virus (HBV) infection. Grade: D

Risk Assessment	The main risk factors for HBV infection include diagnosis with a sexually transmitted disease, intravenous drug use, sexual contact with multiple partners, male homosexual activity, and household contact with chronically infected persons. However, screening strategies to identify individuals at high risk have poor predictive value, since 30–40 percent of infected individuals do not have any easily identifiable risk factors.
Screening Tests	Routine screening of the general population for HBV infection is not recommended.
Interventions	Routine hepatitis vaccination has had significant impact in reducing the number of new HBV infections per year, with the greatest decline among children and adolescents. Programs that vaccinate health care workers also reduce the transmission of HBV infection.
Balance of Benefits and Harms	The USPSTF found no evidence that screening the general population for HBV infection improves long-term health outcomes such as cirrhosis, hepatocellular carcinoma, or mortality. The prevalence of HBV infection is low; the majority of infected individuals do not develop chronic infection, cirrhosis, or HBV-related liver disease. Potential harms of screening include labeling, although there is limited evidence to determine the magnitude of this harm. As a result, the USPSTF concluded that the potential harms of screening for HBV infection in the general population are likely to exceed any potential benefits.
Other Relevant USPSTF Recommendations	The USPSTF has made recommendations on screening for hepatitis B infection in pregnant women and screening for hepatitis C virus infection. These recommendations are available at http://www.uspreventiveservicestaskforce.org/.

For a summary of the evidence systematically reviewed in making this recommendation, the full recommendation statement, and supporting documents, please go to http://www.uspreventiveservicestaskforce.org/.

SCREENING FOR HEPATITIS B VIRUS INFECTION IN PREGNANCY

CLINICAL SUMMARY OF U.S. PREVENTIVE SERVICES TASK FORCE RECOMMENDATION

Population	All pregnant women
Recommendation	Screen for hepatitis B virus (HBV) at the first prenatal visit. Grade: A

Screening Tests	Serologic identification of hepatitis B surface antigen (HBsAg). Reported sensitivity and specificity are greater than 98%.
Timing of Screening	Order HBsAg testing at the first prenatal visit. Re-screen women with unknown HBsAg status or new or continuing risk factors at admission to hospital, birth center, or other delivery setting.
Interventions	Administer hepatitis B vaccine and hepatitis B immune globulin to HBV-exposed infants within 12 hours of birth. Refer women who test positive for counseling and medical management. Counseling should include information about how to prevent transmission to sexual partners and household contacts. Reassure patients that breastfeeding is safe for infants who receive appropriate prophylaxis.
Implementation	Establish systems for timely transfer of maternal HBsAg test results to the labor and delivery and newborn medical records.
Other Relevant USPSTF Recommendations	USPSTF recommendations on the screening of pregnant women for other infections, including asymptomatic bacteriuria, bacterial vaginosis, chlamydia, HIV, and syphilis, can be found at http://www.uspreventiveservicestaskforce.org.

For a summary of the evidence systematically reviewed in making these recommendations, the full recommendation statement, and supporting documents, please go to http://www.uspreventiveservicestaskforce.org.

SCREENING FOR HEPATITIS C VIRUS IN ADULTS

CLINICAL SUMMARY OF U.S. PREVENTIVE SERVICES TASK FORCE RECOMMENDATION

Population	Asymptomatic adults who are not at increased risk for infection	Adults who are at high risk for infection
Recommendation	Do not screen for hepatitis C virus (HCV) infection. Grade: D	No recommendation. Grade: I Statement (Insufficient Evidence)
Risk Assessment	Established risk factors for HCV infection include current or past intravenous drug use, receiving a blood transfusion before 1990, dialysis, and being a child of an HCV-infected mother. Surrogate markers, such as high-risk sexual behavior (particularly sex with someone infected with HCV) and the use of illegal drugs, such as cocaine or marijuana, have also been associated with increased risk for HCV infection.	
Screening Tests	Initial testing for HCV infection is typically done by enzyme immunoassay.	
Interventions	Although there is good evidence that antiviral therapy improves intermediate outcomes, such as viremia, there is limited evidence that such treatment improves long-term health outcomes. The current treatment regimen is long and costly and is associated with a high patient dropout rate due to adverse effects. As of 2004, there was insufficient evidence that newer treatment regimens for HCV infection, such as pegylated interferon plus ribavirin, improve long-term health outcomes.	
Balance of Benefits and Harms	The prevalence of HCV infection in the general population is low, and most who are infected do not develop cirrhosis or other major negative health outcomes. There is no evidence that screening for HCV infection leads to improved long-term health outcomes, such as decreased cirrhosis, hepatocellular cancer, or mortality. Potential harms of screening include unnecessary biopsies and labeling, although there is limited evidence to determine the magnitude of these harms. As a result, the USPSTF concluded that the potential harms of screening for HCV infection in adults who are not at increased risk for HCV infection are likely to exceed the potential benefits.	The USPSTF found no evidence that screening for HCV infection in adults at high risk leads to improved long-term health outcomes. The proportion of persons infected with HCV who progress to liver disease is uncertain. Potential harms of screening and treatment include labeling, adverse treatment effects, and unnecessary biopsies, although there is limited evidence to determine the magnitude of these harms. As a result, the USPSTF could not determine the balance of benefits and harms of screening for HCV infection in adults at increased risk for infection.
Other Relevant USPSTF Recommendations	The USPSTF has made recommendations on screening for hepatitis B virus infection in the general population and in pregnant women. These recommendations are available at http://www.uspreventiveservicestaskforce.org/.	

For a summary of the evidence systematically reviewed in making this recommendation, the full recommendation statement, and supporting documents, please go to http://www.uspreventiveservicestaskforce.org/.

SCREENING FOR HIGH BLOOD PRESSURE IN ADULTS

CLINICAL SUMMARY OF U.S. PREVENTIVE SERVICES TASK FORCE RECOMMENDATION

Population	Adult general population[1]
Recommendation	**Screen for high blood pressure.** **Grade: A**
Screening Tests	High blood pressure (hypertension) is usually defined in adults as: systolic blood pressure (SBP) of 140 mm Hg or higher, or diastolic blood pressure (DBP) of 90 mm Hg or higher. Due to variability in individual blood pressure measurements, it is recommended that hypertension be diagnosed only after 2 or more elevated readings are obtained on at least 2 visits over a period of 1 to several weeks.
Screening Intervals	The optimal interval for screening adults for hypertension is not known. The Joint National Committee on Prevention, Detection, Evaluation, and Treatment of High Blood Pressure (JNC 7) recommends: • Screening every 2 years with BP <120/80. • Screening every year with SBP of 120-139 mmHg or DBP of 80-90 mmHg.
Treatment	A variety of pharmacological agents are available to treat hypertension. JNC 7 guidelines for treatment of hypertension can be accessed at http://www.nhlbi.nih.gov/guidelines/hypertension/jncintro.htm. The following non-pharmacological therapies are associated with reductions in blood pressure: • Reduction of dietary sodium intake. • Potassium supplementation. • Increased physical activity, weight loss. • Stress management. • Reduction of alcohol intake.
Other Relevant USPSTF Recommendations	Adults with hypertension should be screened for diabetes. Adults should be screened for hyperlipidemia (depending on age, sex, risk factors) and smoking. Clinicians should discuss aspirin chemoprevention with patients at increased risk for cardiovascular disease. These recommendations and related evidence are available at http://www.uspreventiveservicestaskforce.org.

[1]This recommendation applies to adults without known hypertension.

For a summary of the evidence systematically reviewed in making these recommendations, the full recommendation statement, and supporting documents, please go to http://www.uspreventiveservicestaskforce.org.

SCREENING FOR HIV

CLINICAL SUMMARY OF U.S. PREVENTIVE SERVICES TASK FORCE RECOMMENDATION

Population	Adolescents and adults at increased risk for HIV infection	Adolescents and adults who are not at increased risk for HIV infection	Pregnant women
Recommendation	Screen for HIV. Grade: A	No recommendation for or against screening. Grade: C	Screen for HIV. Grade: A
Risk Assessment	A person is considered at increased risk for HIV infection if he/she reports one or more individual risk factors or receives health care in a high-prevalence or high-risk clinical setting. High-risk settings include sexually transmitted infection (STI) clinics, correctional facilities, homeless shelters, tuberculosis clinics, clinics serving men who have sex with men, and adolescent health clinics with a high prevalence of STIs. High-prevalence settings are defined as those known to have a 1% or greater prevalence of infection among the patient population being served. Individual risk for HIV infection is assessed through a careful patient history. Individuals at increased risk include: • Men who have had sex with men after 1975 • Persons having unprotected sex with multiple partners • Persons who are past or present injection drug users • Persons who exchange sex for money or drugs or have sex partners who do • Persons whose past or present sex partners are HIV-infected, bisexual, or injection drug users • Persons being treated for sexually transmitted diseases • Persons with a history of blood transfusion between 1978 and 1985 • Persons who request an HIV test despite reporting no risk factors (since this group is likely to include individuals not willing to disclose high risk behaviors)		
Screening Tests	The standard test for diagnosing HIV infection is the repeatedly reactive enzyme immunoassay, followed by confirmatory western blot or immunofluorescent assay. Rapid HIV antibody testing is also highly accurate, can be performed in 10 to 30 minutes, and when offered at the point of care, is useful for screening high-risk patients who do not receive regular medical care (e.g., those seen in emergency departments), as well as women with unknown HIV status who present in active labor.		
Interventions	Evidence supports the benefit of identifying and treating asymptomatic individuals in immunologically advanced stages of HIV disease (i.e., CD4 cell counts <200 cells/mm³) with highly active antiretroviral therapy (HAART). Appropriate prophylaxis and immunization against certain opportunistic infections have also been shown to be effective interventions for these individuals. Use of HAART can be considered for asymptomatic individuals who are in an earlier stage of disease but at high risk for disease progression (i.e., CD4 cell count <350 cells/mm³ or viral load >100,000 copies/mL. Recommended regimens of HAART are acceptable to pregnant women and lead to significantly reduced rates of mother-to-child transmission. Early detection of maternal HIV infection also allows for discussion of elective cesarean section and avoidance of breastfeeding, both of which are associated with lower HIV transmission rates.		
Balance of Benefits and Harms	The USPSTF found good evidence that screening accurately detects HIV infection and that appropriately timed interventions, particularly HAART, lead to improved health outcomes for many of those screened. False-positive test results are rare, and most adverse events associated with treatment, including metabolic disturbances with an increased risk for cardiovascular events, may be ameliorated by changes in regimen. The USPSTF concluded that the benefits of screening individuals at increased risk substantially outweigh potential harms.	The USPSTF found fair evidence that screening individuals who are not known to be at increased risk for HIV can detect additional individuals with HIV, and good evidence that appropriately timed interventions lead to improved health outcomes for some of these individuals. However, the yield of screening persons without risk factors would be low, and there are potential harms of screening. The USPSTF concluded that the benefit of screening individuals without risk factors for HIV is too small relative to the potential harms to justify a general recommendation.	The USPSTF found good evidence that screening accurately detects HIV infection in pregnant women, and fair evidence that prenatal counseling and voluntary testing increases the proportion of HIV-infected women who are diagnosed and treated before delivery. There is no evidence of fetal anomalies or other clinically important fetal harm associated with currently recommended antiretroviral regimens (except for efavirenz). Serious or fatal maternal events are rare using currently recommended combination therapies. The USPSTF concluded that the benefits of screening all pregnant women substantially outweigh the potential harms.
Other Relevant USPSTF Recommendations	The USPSTF has made recommendations on screening and counseling for other sexually transmitted infections. These recommendations are available at http://www.uspreventiveservicestaskforce.org/.		

For a summary of the evidence systematically reviewed in making this recommendation, the full recommendation statement, and supporting documents, please go to http://www.uspreventiveservicestaskforce.org/.

HORMONE REPLACEMENT THERAPY FOR THE PREVENTION OF CHRONIC CONDITIONS IN POSTMENOPAUSAL WOMEN

CLINICAL SUMMARY OF U.S. PREVENTIVE SERVICES TASK FORCE RECOMMENDATION

Population	Postmenopausal women	Postmenopausal women who have had a hysterectomy
Recommendation	Do not use combined estrogen and progestin for the prevention of chronic conditions. Grade: D	Do not use unopposed estrogen for the prevention of chronic conditions. Grade: D
Risk Assessment	The probability that a menopausal woman will develop various chronic diseases during her lifetime is estimated to be: • 46% for coronary heart disease • 20% for stroke • 15% for hip fracture • 10% for breast cancer • 2.6% for endometrial cancer	
Preventive Medication	• Combined estrogen-progestin reduces the risk for fractures and may possibly decrease colorectal cancer risk, but it has no beneficial effect on coronary heart disease. • Combined estrogen-progestin increases the risk for stroke, breast cancer, dementia and lower global cognitive function, venous thromboembolism, and cholecystitis. • There is not enough evidence to determine the effects of hormone therapy on the incidence of ovarian cancer, mortality from breast cancer or coronary heart disease, or all-cause mortality. • Evidence about the effects of different dosages, types, and delivery modes of hormone therapy remains insufficient.	• Estrogen alone decreases a woman's risk for fractures, but it has no beneficial effect on coronary heart disease. • Estrogen alone increases the risk for stroke, dementia and lower global cognitive function, and thromboembolism. • The evidence is insufficient to determine the effects of unopposed estrogen on the incidence of breast cancer, ovarian cancer, or colorectal cancer, as well as breast cancer mortality or all-cause mortality.
Balance of Benefits and Harms	Overall, the harmful effects of combined estrogen and progestin are likely to exceed the benefits of chronic disease prevention for most women.	Overall, the harmful effects of unopposed estrogen are likely to exceed the chronic disease prevention benefits in most women.
Clinical Considerations	The balance of benefits and harms for a woman will be influenced by her personal preferences, her risks for specific chronic diseases, and the presence of menopausal symptoms. A shared decisionmaking approach to preventing chronic diseases in perimenopausal and postmenopausal women involves consideration of individual risk factors and preferences in selecting effective interventions for reducing the risks for fracture, heart disease, and cancer.	
Other Relevant USPSTF Recommendations	Other USPSTF recommendations for prevention of chronic diseases (screening for osteoporosis, high blood pressure, lipid disorders, breast cancer, and colorectal cancer and counseling to prevent tobacco use) are available at http://www.uspreventiveservicestaskforce.org/.	

For a summary of the evidence systematically reviewed in making this recommendation, the full recommendation statement, and supporting documents, please go to http://www.uspreventiveservicestaskforce.org/.

SCREENING FOR ILLICIT DRUG USE

CLINICAL SUMMARY OF U.S. PREVENTIVE SERVICES TASK FORCE RECOMMENDATION

Population	Adolescents, adults, and pregnant women not previously identified as users of illicit drugs
Recommendation	No recommendation. Grade I: (Insufficient Evidence)
Screening Tests	Toxicologic tests of blood or urine can provide objective evidence of drug use, but do not distinguish occasional users from impaired drug users. Valid and reliable standardized questionnaires are available to screen adolescents and adults for drug use or misuse. There is insufficient evidence to evaluate the clinical utility of these instruments when widely applied in primary care settings.
Balance of Benefits and Harms	The USPSTF concludes that for adolescents, adults, and pregnant women, the evidence is insufficient to determine the benefits and harms of screening for illicit drug use.
Suggestions for Practice	Clinicians should be alert to the signs and symptoms of illicit drug use in patients.
Treatment	More evidence is needed on the effectiveness of primary care office-based treatments for illicit drug use/dependence.
Other Relevant USPSTF Recommendations	The USPSTF recommendation for screening and counseling interventions to reduce alcohol misuse by adults and pregnant women can be found at http://www.uspreventiveservicestaskforce.org/uspstf/uspsdrin.htm.

For a summary of the evidence systematically reviewed in making these recommendations, the full recommendation statement, and supporting documents, please go to http://www.uspreventiveservicestaskforce.org.

38

SCREENING FOR IMPAIRED VISUAL ACUITY IN OLDER ADULTS[1]

CLINICAL SUMMARY OF U.S. PREVENTIVE SERVICES TASK FORCE

Population	Adults age 65 and older
Recommendation	No recommendation. Grade: I (Insufficient Evidence)
Risk Assessment	Older age is an important risk factor for most types of visual impairment. Additional risk factors include: • Smoking, alcohol use, exposure to ultraviolet light, diabetes, corticosteroids, and black race (for cataracts). • Smoking, family history, and white race (for age-related macular degeneration).
Screening Tests	Visual acuity testing (for example, the Snellen eye chart) is the usual method for screening for impairment of visual acuity in the primary care setting. Screening questions are not as accurate as a visual acuity test.
Balance of Benefits and Harms	There is no direct evidence that screening for vision impairment in older adults in primary care settings is associated with improved clinical outcomes. There is evidence that early treatment of refractive error, cataracts, and age-related macular degeneration may lead to harms that are small. The magnitude of net benefit for screening cannot be calculated because of a lack of evidence.
Other Relevant USPSTF Recommendations	Recommendations on screening for glaucoma and on screening for hearing loss in older adults can be accessed at http://www.uspreventiveservicestaskforce.org.

[1]This recommendation does not cover screening for glaucoma.

For a summary of the evidence systematically reviewed in making these recommendations, the full recommendation statement, and supporting documents, please go to http://www.uspreventiveservicestaskforce.org.

SCREENING FOR LIPID DISORDERS IN ADULTS

CLINICAL SUMMARY OF U.S. PREVENTIVE SERVICES TASK FORCE RECOMMENDATION

Population	• Men age 35 years and older • Women age 45 years and older who are at increased risk for coronary heart disease (CHD)	• Men ages 20 to 35 years who are at increased risk for CHD • Women ages 20 to 45 years who are at increased risk for CHD	• Men ages 20 to 35 years • Women age 20 years and older who are not at increased risk for CHD
Recommendation	Screen for lipid disorders. Grade: A	Screen for lipid disorders. Grade: B	No recommendation for or against screening Grade: C
Risk Assessment	Consideration of lipid levels along with other risk factors allows for an accurate estimation of CHD risk. Risk factors for CHD include diabetes, history of previous CHD or atherosclerosis, family history of cardiovascular disease, tobacco use, hypertension, and obesity (body mass index ≥30 kg/m²).		
Screening Tests	The preferred screening tests for dyslipidemia are measuring serum lipid (total cholesterol, high-density and low-density lipoprotein cholesterol) levels in non-fasting or fasting samples. Abnormal screening results should be confirmed by a repeated sample on a separate occasion, and the average of both results should be used for risk assessment.		
Timing of Screening	The optimal interval for screening is uncertain. Reasonable options include every 5 years, shorter intervals for people who have lipid levels close to those warranting therapy, and longer intervals for those not at increased risk who have had repeatedly normal lipid levels. An age at which to stop screening has not been established. Screening may be appropriate in older people who have never been screened; repeated screening is less important in older people because lipid levels are less likely to increase after age 65 years.		
Interventions	Drug therapy is usually more effective than diet alone in improving lipid profiles, but choice of treatment should consider overall risk, costs of treatment, and patient preferences. Guidelines for treating lipid disorders are available from the National Cholesterol Education Program of the National Institutes of Health (http://www.nhlbi.nih.gov/about/ncep/).		
Balance of Benefits and Harms	The benefits of screening for and treating lipid disorders in men age 35 and older and women age 45 and older at increased risk for CHD substantially outweigh the potential harms.	The benefits of screening for and treating lipid disorders in young adults at increased risk for CHD moderately outweigh the potential harms.	The net benefits of screening for lipid disorders in young adults not at increased risk for CHD are not sufficient to make a general recommendation.
Other Relevant USPSTF Recommendations	The USPSTF has made recommendations on screening for lipid disorders in children and screening for carotid artery stenosis, coronary heart disease, high blood pressure, and peripheral arterial disease. These recommendations are available at http://www.uspreventiveservicestaskforce.org/.		

For a summary of the evidence systematically reviewed in making this recommendation, the full recommendation statement, and supporting documents, please go to http://www.uspreventiveservicestaskforce.org/.

SCREENING FOR LUNG CANCER

CLINICAL SUMMARY OF U.S. PREVENTIVE SERVICES TASK FORCE RECOMMENDATION

Population	Asymptomatic persons
Recommendation	No recommendation. Grade: I (Insufficient Evidence)
Risk Assessment	Cigarette smoking is the major risk factor for lung cancer. Other risk factors include family history, chronic obstructive pulmonary disease, idiopathic pulmonary fibrosis, environmental radon exposure, passive smoking, asbestos exposure, and certain occupational exposures.
Screening Tests	Screening with low dose computerized tomography, chest x-ray, or sputum cytology can detect lung cancer at earlier stages; however, as of 2004, there is insufficient evidence that any screening strategy for lung cancer decreases mortality.
Balance of Benefits and Harms	As of 2004, the benefit of screening for lung cancer has not been established in any group, including asymptomatic high-risk populations such as older smokers. The balance of Benefits and Harms becomes increasingly unfavorable for persons at lower risk, such as nonsmokers. Because of the invasive nature of diagnostic testing and the possibility of a high number of false-positive results in certain populations, there is potential for significant harms from screening. Therefore, the USPSTF could not determine the balance between the benefits and harms of screening for lung cancer.
Other Relevant USPSTF Recommendations	The USPSTF has made recommendations on screening for many other types of cancer. These recommendations are available at http://www.uspreventiveservicestaskforce.org/.

For a summary of the evidence systematically reviewed in making this recommendation, the full recommendation statement, and supporting documents, please go to http://www.uspreventiveservicestaskforce.org/.

PRIMARY CARE COUNSELING FOR PROPER USE OF MOTOR VEHICLE OCCUPANT RESTRAINTS

CLINICAL SUMMARY OF U.S. PREVENTIVE SERVICES TASK FORCE RECOMMENDATIONS

Population	General primary care population
Recommendation	No recommendation. Grade: I (Insufficient Evidence)

Interventions	There is good evidence that community and public health interventions, including legislation, law enforcement campaigns, car seat distribution campaigns, media campaigns, and other community-based interventions, are effective in improving the proper use of car seats, booster seats, and seat belts.
Suggestions for Practice	Current evidence is insufficient to assess the incremental benefit of counseling in primary care settings, beyond increases related to other interventions, in improving rates of proper use of motor vehicle occupant restraints. Linkages between primary care and community interventions are critical for improving proper car seat, booster seat, and seat belt use.
Relevant Recommendations from the *Guide to Community Preventive Services*	The Community Preventive Services Task Force has reviewed evidence of the effectiveness of selected population-based interventions to reduce motor vehicle occupant injuries, focusing on three strategic areas: • Increasing the proper use of child safety seats. • Increasing the use of safety belts. • Reducing alcohol-impaired driving. Multiple interventions in these areas have been recommended. Recommendations can be accessed at http://www.thecommunityguide.org/mvoi/

For a summary of the evidence systematically reviewed in making these recommendations, the full recommendation statement, and supporting documents, please go to http://www.uspreventiveservicestaskforce.org.

SCREENING FOR ORAL CANCER

CLINICAL SUMMARY OF U.S. PREVENTIVE SERVICES TASK FORCE RECOMMENDATION

Population	Asymptomatic adults
Recommendation	No recommendation. Grade: I Statement (Insufficient Evidence)

Risk Assessment	Tobacco use in all forms is the biggest risk factor for oral cancer. Alcohol abuse combined with tobacco use increases risk. Clinicians should be alert to the possibility of oral cancer when treating patients who use tobacco or alcohol.
Screening Tests	Direct inspection and palpation of the oral cavity is the most commonly recommended method of screening for oral cancer, although there are little data on the sensitivity and specificity of this method. Screening techniques other than inspection and palpation are being evaluated but are still experimental.
Interventions	Patients should be encouraged to not use tobacco and to limit alcohol use in order to decrease their risk for oral cancer, as well as for heart disease, stroke, lung cancer, and cirrhosis.
Balance of Benefits and Harms	There is no good-quality evidence that screening for oral cancer leads to improved health outcomes for either high-risk adults (i.e., adults older than age 50 years who use tobacco) or average-risk adults in the general population. It is unlikely that controlled trials of screening for oral cancer will ever be conducted in the general population because of the very low incidence of oral cancer in the United States. There is also no evidence of the harms of screening. As a result, the USPSTF could not determine the balance between the benefits and harms of screening for oral cancer.
Other Relevant USPSTF Recommendations	The USPSTF has made recommendations on screening for many other types of cancer. These recommendations are available at http://www.uspreventiveservicestaskforce.org/.

For a summary of the evidence systematically reviewed in making this recommendation, the full recommendation statement, and supporting documents, please go to http://www.uspreventiveservicestaskforce.org/.

43

SCREENING FOR OSTEOPOROSIS

CLINICAL SUMMARY OF U.S. PREVENTIVE SERVICES TASK FORCE RECOMMENDATION

Population	Women age ≥65 years without previous known fractures or secondary causes of osteoporosis	Women age <65 years whose 10-year fracture risk is equal to or greater than that of a 65-year-old white woman without additional risk factors	Men without previous known fractures or secondary causes of osteoporosis
Recommendation	Screen for osteoporosis. Grade: B		No recommendation. Grade: I (Insufficient Evidence)

Risk Assessment	As many as 1 in 2 postmenopausal women and 1 in 5 older men are at risk for an osteoporosis-related fracture. Osteoporosis is common in all racial groups but is most common in white persons. Rates of osteoporosis increase with age. Elderly people are particularly susceptible to fractures. According to the FRAX fracture risk assessment tool, available at http://www.shef.ac.uk/FRAX/, the 10-year fracture risk in a 65-year-old white woman without additional risk factors is 9.3%.
Screening Tests	Current diagnostic and treatment criteria rely on dual-energy x-ray absorptiometry of the hip and lumbar spine.
Timing of Screening	Evidence is lacking about optimal intervals for repeated screening.
Intervention	In addition to adequate calcium and vitamin D intake and weight-bearing exercise, multiple U.S. Food and Drug Administration-approved therapies reduce fracture risk in women with low bone mineral density and no previous fractures, including bisphosphonates, parathyroid hormone, raloxifene, and estrogen. The choice of treatment should take into account the patient's clinical situation and the tradeoff between benefits and harms. Clinicians should provide education about how to minimize drug side effects.
Suggestions for Practice Regarding the I Statement for Men	Clinicians should consider: • potential preventable burden: increasing because of the aging of the U.S. population • potential harms: likely to be small, mostly opportunity costs • current practice: routine screening of men not widespread • costs: additional scanners required to screen sizeable populations Men most likely to benefit from screening have a 10-year risk for osteoporotic fracture equal to or greater than that of a 65-year-old white woman without risk factors. However, current evidence is insufficient to assess the balance of benefits and harms of screening for osteoporosis in men.

For a summary of the evidence systematically reviewed in making these recommendations, the full recommendation statement, and supporting documents, please go to http://www.uspreventiveservicestaskforce.org.

SCREENING FOR OVARIAN CANCER

CLINICAL SUMMARY OF U.S. PREVENTIVE SERVICES TASK FORCE RECOMMENDATION

Population	Adult women
Recommendation	Do not screen for ovarian cancer. Grade: D

Risk Assessment	The following risk factors are associated with ovarian cancer: family history, carrying the *BRCA1* or *BRCA2* gene mutations, and possibly taking estrogen supplementation for postmenopausal chronic conditions.
Screening Tests	Screening with serum CA-125 level or transvaginal ultrasonography may detect ovarian cancer at earlier stages than in the absence of screening; however, earlier detection likely has a small effect, at best, on mortality from ovarian cancer. Also, because there is a low incidence of ovarian cancer in the general population, screening for ovarian cancer is likely to have a relatively low yield.
Balance of Benefits and Harms	Because of the low prevalence of ovarian cancer and the invasive nature of diagnostic testing after a positive screening test, there is fair evidence that screening could likely lead to important harms. Therefore, the potential harms of screening for ovarian cancer outweigh the potential benefits.
Other Relevant USPSTF Recommendations	The USPSTF has also made recommendations on genetic risk assessment and *BRCA* mutation testing for ovarian and breast cancer susceptibility, as well as screening for breast cancer and cervical cancer. These recommendations are available at http://www.uspreventiveservicestaskforce.org/.

For a summary of the evidence systematically reviewed in making this recommendation, the full recommendation statement, and supporting documents, please go to http://www.uspreventiveservicestaskforce.org/.

SCREENING FOR PANCREATIC CANCER

CLINICAL SUMMARY OF U.S. PREVENTIVE SERVICES TASK FORCE RECOMMENDATION

Population	Asymptomatic adults
Recommendation	Do not screen for pancreatic cancer. Grade: D

Risk Assessment	Persons with hereditary pancreatitis may have a higher lifetime risk for developing pancreatic cancer. However, the USPSTF did not review the effectiveness of screening these patients.
Balance of Benefits and Harms	The USPSTF found no evidence that screening for pancreatic cancer is effective in reducing mortality. There is a potential for significant harm due to the very low prevalence of pancreatic cancer, limited accuracy of available screening tests, the invasive nature of diagnostic tests, and the poor outcomes of treatment. As a result, the USPSTF concluded that the harms of screening for pancreatic cancer exceed any potential benefits.
Other Relevant USPSTF Recommendations	The USPSTF has made recommendations on screening for many types of cancer. These recommendations are available at http://www.uspreventiveservicestaskforce.org/.

For a summary of the evidence systematically reviewed in making this recommendation, the full recommendation statement, and supporting documents, please go to http://www.uspreventiveservicestaskforce.org/.

SCREENING FOR PERIPHERAL ARTERIAL DISEASE

CLINICAL SUMMARY OF U.S. PREVENTIVE SERVICES TASK FORCE RECOMMENDATION

Population	Asymptomatic adults
Recommendation	Do not screen for peripheral arterial disease (PAD). Grade: D

Risk Assessment	Risk factors associated with PAD include older age, cigarette smoking, diabetes mellitus, hypercholesterolemia, hypertension, and possibly genetic factors.
Screening Tests	Ankle brachial index (ABI) is a simple and accurate noninvasive test for the screening and diagnosis of PAD. The ABI has demonstrated better accuracy than other methods of screening, including history taking, questionnaires, and palpation of peripheral pulses. An ABI value of less than 0.90 (95% sensitive and specific for angiographic PAD) is strongly associated with limitations in lower extremity functioning and physical activity tolerance.
Interventions	Smoking cessation and physical activity training also increase maximal walking distance among men with early PAD.
Balance of Benefits and Harms	Screening for PAD in asymptomatic adults in the general population has few or no benefits, because the prevalence of PAD in this group is low and because there is little evidence that treatment of PAD at this asymptomatic stage of disease, beyond treatment based on standard cardiovascular risk assessment, improves health outcomes. Screening asymptomatic adults with the ankle brachial index could lead to some small degree of harm, including false-positive results and unnecessary workups. Therefore, the harms of routine screening for PAD exceed the benefits for asymptomatic adults.
Other Relevant USPSTF Recommendations	The USPSTF has made recommendations on screening for carotid artery stenosis, coronary heart disease, high blood pressure, and lipid disorders. These recommendations are available at http://www.uspreventiveservicestaskforce.org/.

For a summary of the evidence systematically reviewed in making this recommendation, the full recommendation statement, and supporting documents, please go to http://www.uspreventiveservicestaskforce.org/.

SCREENING FOR Rh (D) INCOMPATIBILITY

CLINICAL SUMMARY OF U.S. PREVENTIVE SERVICES TASK FORCE RECOMMENDATION

Population	Pregnant women presenting at the first visit for prenatal care	Unsensitized Rh (D)-negative women at 24–28 weeks' gestation
Recommendation	Perform Rh (D) blood typing and antibody testing. Grade: A	Repeat Rh (D) blood typing and antibody testing. Grade: B
Screening Tests	Rh (D) blood typing and antibody testing prevents maternal sensitization and improves outcomes for newborns.	
Timing of Screening	Repeated antibody testing in unsensitized Rh (D)-negative women, unless the father is also known to be Rh (D)-negative, provides additional benefit over a single test at the first prenatal visit.	
Interventions	• Administration of a full (300 μg) dose of Rh (D) immunoglobulin is recommended for all unsensitized Rh (D)-negative women after repeated antibody testing at 24–28 weeks' gestation. • If an Rh (D)-positive or weakly Rh (D)-positive infant is delivered, a dose of Rh (D) immunoglobulin should be repeated postpartum, preferably within 72 hours after delivery. • Unless the biological father is known to be Rh (D)-negative, a full dose of Rh (D) immunoglobulin is recommended for all unsensitized Rh (D)-negative women after amniocentesis and after induced or spontaneous abortion; however, if the pregnancy is less than 13 weeks, a 50 μg dose is sufficient.	
Balance of Benefits and Harms	The benefits of Rh (D) blood typing and antibody testing at the first prenatal visit substantially outweigh any potential harms.	The benefits of repeated testing substantially outweigh any potential harms.
Other Relevant USPSTF Recommendations	The USPSTF has made recommendations on many types of obstetric screenings. These recommendations are available at http://www.uspreventiveservicestaskforce.org/.	

For a summary of the evidence systematically reviewed in making this recommendation, the full recommendation statement, and supporting documents, please go to http://www.uspreventiveservicestaskforce.org/.

BEHAVIORAL COUNSELING TO PREVENT SEXUALLY TRANSMITTED INFECTIONS

CLINICAL SUMMARY OF U.S. PREVENTIVE SERVICES TASK FORCE RECOMMENDATION

Population	All sexually active adolescents	Adults at increased risk for STIs	Non-sexually-active adolescents and adults not at increased risk for STIs
Recommendation	Offer high-intensity counseling. Grade: B	Offer high-intensity counseling. Grade: B	No recommendation. Grade: I (Insufficient Evidence)
Risk Assessment	All sexually active adolescents are at increased risk for STIs and should be offered counseling. Adults should be considered at increased risk and offered counseling if they have: • Current STIs or have had an STI within the past year. • Multiple sexual partners. In communities or populations with high rates of STIs, all sexually active patients in non-monogamous relationships may be considered at increased risk.		
Interventions	Characteristics of successful high-intensity counseling interventions: • Multiple sessions of counseling. • Frequently delivered in group settings.		
Suggestions for Practice	High-intensity counseling may be delivered in primary care settings, or in other sectors of the health system and community settings after referral. Delivery of this service may be greatly improved by strong linkages between the primary care setting and community.		Evidence is limited regarding counseling for adolescents who are not sexually active. Intensive counseling for all adolescents in order to reach those who are at risk but have not been appropriately identified is not supported by current evidence. Evidence is lacking regarding the effectiveness of counseling for adults not at increased risk for STIs.
Other Relevant USPSTF Recommendations	USPSTF recommendations on screening for chlamydial infection, gonorrhea, genital herpes, hepatitis B, hepatitis C, HIV, and syphilis can be found at http://www.uspreventiveservicestaskforce.org.		

Abbreviation: STI = Sexually Transmitted Infection

For a summary of the evidence systematically reviewed in making these recommendations, the full recommendation statement, and supporting documents, please go to http://www.uspreventiveservicestaskforce.org.

SCREENING FOR SKIN CANCER

CLINICAL SUMMARY OF U.S. PREVENTIVE SERVICES TASK FORCE RECOMMENDATION

Population	Adult general population[1]
Recommendation	No recommendation. Grade: I (Insufficient Evidence)
Risk Assessment	Skin cancer risks: family history of skin cancer, considerable history of sun exposure and sunburn. Groups at increased risk for melanoma: • Fair-skinned men and women over the age of 65 years. • Patients with atypical moles. • Patients with more than 50 moles.
Screening Tests	There is insufficient evidence to assess the balance of benefits and harms of whole body skin examination by a clinician or patient skin self-examination for the early detection of skin cancer.
Screening Intervals	Not applicable.
Suggestions for Practice	Clinicians should remain alert for skin lesions with malignant features that are noted while performing physical examinations for other purposes. Features associated with increased risk for malignancy include: asymmetry, border irregularity, color variability, diameter >6mm ("A," "B," "C," "D"), or rapidly changing lesions. Suspicious lesions should be biopsied.
Other Relevant Recommendations from the USPSTF and the Community Preventive Services Task Force	The USPSTF has reviewed the evidence for counseling to prevent skin cancer. The recommendation statement and supporting documents can be accessed at http://www.uspreventiveservicestaskforce.org. The Community Preventive Services Task Force has reviewed the evidence on public health interventions to reduce skin cancer. The recommendations can be accessed at http://www.thecommunityguide.org.

[1]The USPSTF does not examine outcomes related to surveillance of patients with familial syndromes, such as familial atypical mole and melanoma (FAM-M) syndrome.

For a summary of the evidence systematically reviewed in making these recommendations, the full recommendation statement, and supporting documents, please go to http://www.uspreventiveservicestaskforce.org.

SCREENING FOR SUICIDE RISK

CLINICAL SUMMARY OF U.S. PREVENTIVE SERVICES TASK FORCE RECOMMENDATION

Population	General population
Recommendation	No recommendation. Grade: I (Insufficient Evidence)
Risk Assessment	The strongest risk factors for attempted suicide include mood disorders or other mental disorders, comorbid substance abuse disorders, history of deliberate self-harm, and a history of suicide attempts. Deliberate self-harm refers to intentionally initiated acts of self-harm with a nonfatal outcome (including self-poisoning and self-injury). Suicide risk is assessed along a continuum ranging from suicidal ideation alone (relatively less severe) to suicidal ideation with a plan (more severe). Suicidal ideation with a specific plan of action is associated with a significant risk for attempted suicide.
Screening Tests	There is limited evidence on the accuracy of screening tools to identify suicide risk in the primary care setting, including tools to identify those at high risk. The characteristics of the most commonly used screening instruments (Scale for Suicide Ideation, Scale for Suicide Ideation–Worst, and the Suicidal Ideation Questionnaire) have not been validated to assess suicide risk in primary care settings.
Interventions	There is insufficient evidence to determine if treatment of persons at high risk for suicide reduces suicide attempts or mortality.
Balance of Benefits and Harms	There is no evidence that screening for suicide risk reduces suicide attempts or mortality. There is insufficient evidence to determine if treatment of persons at high risk reduces suicide attempts or mortality. There are no studies that directly address the harms of screening and treatment for suicide risk. As a result, the USPSTF could not determine the balance of benefits and harms of screening for suicide risk in the primary care setting.
Other Relevant USPSTF Recommendations	The USPSTF has also made recommendations on screening for alcohol misuse, depression, and illicit drug use. These recommendations are available at http://www.uspreventiveservicestaskforce.org/.

For a summary of the evidence systematically reviewed in making this recommendation, the full recommendation statement, and supporting documents, please go to http://www.uspreventiveservicestaskforce.org/.

51

SCREENING FOR SYPHILIS INFECTION

CLINICAL SUMMARY OF U.S. PREVENTIVE SERVICES TASK FORCE RECOMMENDATION

Population	Persons at increased risk for syphilis infection	Asymptomatic persons who are not at increased risk for syphilis infection
Recommendation	Screen for syphilis infection. Grade: A	Do not screen for syphilis infection. Grade: D
Risk Assessment	Populations at increased risk for syphilis infection include men who have sex with men and engage in high-risk sexual behavior, commercial sex workers, persons who exchange sex for drugs, and those in adult correctional facilities. Persons diagnosed with other sexually transmitted diseases may be more likely than others to engage in high-risk behavior, placing them at increased risk.	
Screening Tests	Screening for syphilis infection is a two-step process that involves an initial nontreponemal test (Venereal Disease Research Laboratory or Rapid Plasma Reagin), followed by a confirmatory treponemal test (fluorescent treponemal antibody absorbed or *T. pallidum* particle agglutination).	
Timing of Screening	The optimal screening interval in average- and high-risk persons has not been determined.	
Interventions	Preferred treatment consists of antibiotic therapy with parenterally administered penicillin G.	
Balance of Benefits and Harms	Screening may result in potential harms (such as false-positive results, unnecessary anxiety to the patient, and harms of antibiotic use). However, the benefits of screening persons at increased risk for syphilis infection substantially outweigh the potential harms.	Given the low incidence of infection in the general population and the consequent low yield of such screening, the potential harms of screening (i.e., opportunity costs, false-positive tests, and labeling) in a low-incident population outweigh the benefits.
Other Relevant USPSTF Recommendations	The USPSTF has made other recommendations on screening for sexually transmitted infections, including screening for syphilis infection in pregnant women. These recommendations are available at http://www.uspreventiveservicestaskforce.org/.	

For a summary of the evidence systematically reviewed in making this recommendation, the full recommendation statement, and supporting documents, please go to http://www.uspreventiveservicestaskforce.org/.

SCREENING FOR SYPHILIS INFECTION IN PREGNANCY

CLINICAL SUMMARY OF U.S. PREVENTIVE SERVICES TASK FORCE RECOMMENDATION

Population	All pregnant women
Recommendation	Screen for syphilis infection. Grade: A
Screening Tests	Nontreponemal tests commonly used for initial screening include: • Venereal Disease Research Laboratory (VDRL) • Rapid Plasma Reagin (RPR) Confirmatory tests include: • Fluorescent treponemal antibody absorbed (FTA-ABS) • *Treponema pallidum* particle agglutination (TPPA)
Timing of Screening	Test all pregnant women at the first prenatal visit.
Other Clinical Considerations	Most organizations recommend testing high-risk women again during the third trimester and at delivery. Groups at increased risk include: • Uninsured women • Women living in poverty • Sex workers • Illicit drug users • Those diagnosed with other sexually transmitted infections (STIs) • Other women living in communities with high syphilis morbidity Prevalence is higher in southern U.S. and in metropolitan areas and in Hispanic and African American populations.
Interventions	The Centers for Disease Control and Prevention (CDC) recommends treatment with parenteral benzathine penicillin G. Women with penicillin allergies should be desensitized and treated with penicillin. Consult the CDC for the most up-to-date recommendations: http://www.cdc.gov/std/treatment/.
Other Relevant USPSTF Recommendations	Recommendations on screening for other STIs, and on counseling for STIs, can be found at http://www.uspreventiveservicestaskforce.org.

For a summary of the evidence systematically reviewed in making these recommendations, the full recommendation statement, and supporting documents, please go to http://www.uspreventiveservicestaskforce.org.

SCREENING FOR TESTICULAR CANCER

CLINICAL SUMMARY OF U.S. PREVENTIVE SERVICES TASK FORCE RECOMMENDATION

Population	Adolescent and adult males
Recommendation	Do not screen. Grade: D

Screening Tests	There is inadequate evidence that screening asymptomatic patients by means of self-examination or clinician examination has greater yield or accuracy for detecting testicular cancer at more curable stages.
Interventions	Management of testicular cancer consists of orchiectomy and may include other surgery, radiation therapy, or chemotherapy, depending on stage and tumor type. Regardless of disease stage, over 90% of all newly diagnosed cases of testicular cancer will be cured.
Balance of Benefits and Harms	Screening by self-examination or clinician examination is unlikely to offer meaningful health benefits, given the very low incidence and high cure rate of even advanced testicular cancer. Potential harms include false-positive results, anxiety, and harms from diagnostic tests or procedures.
Other Relevant USPSTF Recommendations	Recommendations on screening for other types of cancer can be found at http://www.uspreventiveservicestaskforce.org.

For a summary of the evidence systematically reviewed in making these recommendations, the full recommendation statement, and supporting documents, please go to http://www.uspreventiveservicestaskforce.org.

SCREENING FOR THYROID DISEASE

CLINICAL SUMMARY OF U.S. PREVENTIVE SERVICES TASK FORCE RECOMMENDATION

Population	Asymptomatic adults
Recommendation	No recommendation. Grade: I Statement (Insufficient Evidence)

Risk Assessment	People at higher risk for thyroid dysfunction include the elderly, postpartum women, persons with high levels of radiation exposure (>20 mGy), and patients with Down syndrome.
Screening Tests	Screening for thyroid dysfunction can be performed using the medical history, physical examination, or any of several serum thyroid function tests. Thyroid stimulating hormone (TSH) is usually recommended because it can detect abnormalities before other tests become abnormal.
Interventions	A potential benefit of treating subclinical thyroid disease is to prevent the spontaneous development of overt hypothyroidism or hyperthyroidism, but this potential benefit has not been well studied in clinical trials as of 2004.
Balance of Benefits and Harms	There is fair evidence that the TSH test can detect subclinical thyroid disease in persons without symptoms of thyroid dysfunction, but poor evidence that treatment improves clinically important outcomes in adults with screen-detected thyroid disease. There is the potential for harm caused by false-positive screening tests; however, the magnitude of harm is not known. There is good evidence that overtreatment with levothyroxine occurs in a substantial proportion of patients, but the long-term harmful effects of overtreatment are not known. As a result, the USPSTF could not determine the balance of benefits and harms of screening asymptomatic adults for thyroid disease.
Other Relevant USPSTF Recommendations	The USPSTF has also made recommendations on screening for diabetes, hemochromatosis, iron deficiency anemia, and obesity. These recommendations are available at http://www.uspreventiveservicestaskforce.org/.

For a summary of the evidence systematically reviewed in making this recommendation, the full recommendation statement, and supporting documents, please go to http://www.uspreventiveservicestaskforce.org/.

COUNSELING AND INTERVENTIONS TO PREVENT TOBACCO USE AND TOBACCO-CAUSED DISEASE IN ADULTS AND PREGNANT WOMEN

CLINICAL SUMMARY OF U.S. PREVENTIVE SERVICES TASK FORCE RECOMMENDATION

Population	Adults age ≥ 18 years	Pregnant women of any age
Recommendation	Ask about tobacco use. Provide tobacco cessation interventions to those who use tobacco products. Grade: A	Ask about tobacco use. Provide augmented pregnancy-tailored counseling for women who smoke. Grade: A
Counseling	The "5-A" framework provides a useful counseling strategy: 1. **Ask** about tobacco use. 2. **Advise** to quit through clear personalized messages. 3. **Assess** willingness to quit. 4. **Assist** to quit. 5. **Arrange** follow-up and support. Intensity of counseling matters: brief one-time counseling works; however, longer sessions or multiple sessions are more effective. Telephone counseling "quit lines" also improve cessation rates.	
Pharmacotherapy	Combination therapy with counseling and medications is more effective than either component alone. FDA-approved pharmacotherapy includes nicotine replacement therapy, sustained-release bupropion, and varenicline.	The USPSTF found inadequate evidence to evaluate the safety or efficacy of pharmacotherapy during pregnancy.
Implementation	Successful implementation strategies for primary care practice include: • Instituting a tobacco user identification system. • Promoting clinician intervention through education, resources, and feedback. • Dedicating staff to provide treatment, and assessing the delivery of treatment in staff performance evaluations.	
Other Relevant USPSTF Recommendations	Recommendations on other behavioral counseling topics are available at http://www.uspreventiveservicestaskforce.org.	

Abbreviations: FDA = U.S. Food and Drug Administration; USPSTF = U.S. Preventive Services Task Force

For a summary of the evidence systematically reviewed in making these recommendations, the full recommendation statement, and supporting documents, please go to http://www.uspreventiveservicestaskforce.org.

Recommendations for Children and Adolescents

All clinical summaries in this Guide are abridged recommendations. To see the full recommendation statements and recommendations published after March 2012, go to www.USPreventiveServicesTaskForce.org.

SCREENING FOR ELEVATED BLOOD LEAD LEVELS IN CHILDREN AND PREGNANT WOMEN

CLINICAL SUMMARY OF U.S. PREVENTIVE SERVICES TASK FORCE RECOMMENDATION

Population	Asymptomatic children ages 1 to 5 years who are at increased risk	Asymptomatic children ages 1 to 5 years who are at average risk	Asymptomatic pregnant women
Recommendation	No recommendation. Grade: I (Insufficient Evidence)	Do not screen for elevated blood lead levels. Grade: D	Do not screen for elevated blood lead levels. Grade: D
Risk Assessment	Children younger than age 5 years are at greater risk for elevated blood lead levels and lead toxicity because of increased hand-to-mouth activity, increased lead absorption from the gastrointestinal tract, and the greater vulnerability of the developing central nervous system. Risk factors for increased blood lead levels in children and adults include: minority race/ethnicity; urban residence; low income; low educational attainment; older (pre-1950) housing; recent or ongoing home renovation or remodeling; pica; use of ethnic remedies, certain cosmetics, and exposure to lead-glazed pottery; occupational exposure; and recent immigration. Additional risk factors for pregnant women include alcohol use and smoking.		
Screening Tests	Venous sampling accurately detects elevated blood lead levels. Screening questionnaires may be of value in identifying children at risk for elevated blood lead levels, but should be tailored for and validated in specific communities for clinical use.		
Interventions	Treatment options for elevated blood lead levels include residential lead hazard-control efforts (i.e., counseling and education, dust or paint removal, and soil abatement), chelation, and nutritional interventions. Community-based interventions for the prevention of lead exposure are likely to be more effective, and may be more cost-effective, than office-based screening, treatment, and counseling. Relocating children who do not yet have elevated blood lead levels but who live in settings with high lead exposure may be especially helpful.		
Balance of Benefits and Harms	There is not enough evidence to assess the balance between the potential benefits and harms of routine screening for elevated blood lead levels in children at increased risk.	Given the significant potential harms of treatment and residential lead hazard abatement, and no evidence of treatment benefit, the harms of screening for elevated blood lead levels in children at average risk outweigh the benefits.	Given the significant potential harms of treatment and residential lead hazard abatement, and no evidence of treatment benefit, the harms of screening for elevated blood lead levels in asymptomatic pregnant women outweigh the benefits.

For a summary of the evidence systematically reviewed in making this recommendation, the full recommendation statement, and supporting documents, please go to http://www.uspreventiveservicestaskforce.org/.

SCREENING FOR CONGENITAL HYPOTHYROIDISM

CLINICAL SUMMARY OF U.S. PREVENTIVE SERVICES TASK FORCE RECOMMENDATION

Population	All newborn infants[1]
Recommendation	Screen for congenital hypothyroidism. Grade: A
Screening Tests	Two methods of screening are used most frequently in the United States: • Primary TSH with backup T4. • Primary T4 with backup TSH. Screening for congenital hypothyroidism (CH) is mandated in all 50 states and the District of Columbia. Clinicians should become familiar with the tests used in their area and the limitations of the screening strategies employed.
Timing of Screening	Infants should be tested between 2 and 4 days of age. Infants discharged from hospitals before 48 hours of life should be tested immediately before discharge. Specimens obtained in the first 24-48 hours of age may be falsely elevated for TSH regardless of the screening method used.
Suggestions for Practice	Infants with abnormal screens should receive confirmatory testing and begin appropriate treatment with thyroid hormone replacement within 2 weeks after birth. Children with positive confirmatory testing in whom no permanent cause of CH is found should undergo a 30-day trial of reduced or discontinued thyroid hormone replacement therapy to determine if the hypothyroidism is permanent or transient. This trial of reduced or discontinued therapy should take place at some time after the child reaches 3 years of age.
Other Relevant Recommendations from the USPSTF	Additional USPSTF recommendations regarding screening tests for newborns can be accessed at: http://www.uspreventiveservicestaskforce.org/recommendations.htm#pediatric

[1]This recommendation applies to all infants born in the U.S. Premature, very low birth weight and ill infants may benefit from additional screening. These conditions are associated with decreased sensitivity and specificity of screening tests.

For a summary of the evidence systematically reviewed in making these recommendations, the full recommendation statement, and supporting documents, please go to http://www.uspreventiveservicestaskforce.org.

SCREENING FOR DEVELOPMENTAL DYSPLASIA OF THE HIP

CLINICAL SUMMARY OF U.S. PREVENTIVE SERVICES TASK FORCE RECOMMENDATION

Population	Infants who do not have obvious hip dislocations or other abnormalities evident without screening
Recommendation	No recommendation. Grade: I (Insufficient Evidence)

Risk Assessment	Risk factors for developmental dysplasia of the hip include female sex, family history, breech positioning, and in utero postural deformities. However, the majority of cases of developmental dysplasia of the hip have no identifiable risk factors.
Screening Tests	Screening tests for developmental dysplasia of the hip have limited accuracy. The most common methods of screening are serial physical examinations of the hip and lower extremities, using the Barlow and Ortolani procedures, and ultrasonography.
Interventions	Treatments for developmental dysplasia of the hip include both nonsurgical and surgical options. Nonsurgical treatment with abduction devices is used as early treatment and includes the commonly prescribed Pavlik method. Surgical intervention is used when the dysplasia is severe or diagnosed late, or after an unsuccessful trial of nonsurgical treatment. Avascular necrosis of the hip is the most common and most severe potential harm of both surgical and nonsurgical interventions, and can result in growth arrest of the hip and eventual joint destruction, with significant disability.
Balance of Benefits and Harms	The USPSTF was unable to assess the balance of benefits and harms of screening for developmental dysplasia of the hip due to insufficient evidence. There are concerns about the potential harms associated with treatment of infants identified by routine screening.
Other Relevant USPSTF Recommendations	The USPSTF has made recommendations on screening for hyperbilirubinemia, phenylketonuria, sickle cell disease, congenital hypothyroidism, and hearing loss in newborns. These recommendations are available at http://www.uspreventiveservicestaskforce.org/.

For a summary of the evidence systematically reviewed in making this recommendation, the full recommendation statement, and supporting documents, please go to http://www.uspreventiveservicestaskforce.org/.

OCULAR PROPHYLAXIS FOR GONOCOCCAL OPHTHALMIA NEONATORUM

CLINICAL SUMMARY OF U.S. PREVENTIVE SERVICES TASK FORCE REAFFIRMATION RECOMMENDATION

Population	All newborn infants
Recommendation	Provide prophylactic ocular topical medication for the prevention of gonococcal ophthalmia neonatorum. Grade: A

Risk Assessment	All newborns should receive prophylaxis. However, some newborns are at increased risk, including those with a maternal history of no prenatal care, sexually transmitted infections, or substance abuse.
Preventive Interventions	Preventive medications include 0.5% erythromycin ophthalmic ointment, 1.0% solution of silver nitrate, and 1.0% tetracycline ointment. All are considered equally effective; however, the latter two are no longer available in the United States.
Timing of Intervention	Within 24 hours after birth.
Other Relevant USPSTF Recommendations	Several recommendations on screening and counseling for infectious diseases and perinatal care can be found at: http://www.uspreventiveservicestaskforce.org.

For a summary of the evidence systematically reviewed in making these recommendations, the full recommendation statement, and supporting documents, please go to http://www.uspreventiveservicestaskforce.org.

UNIVERSAL SCREENING FOR HEARING LOSS IN NEWBORNS

CLINICAL SUMMARY OF U.S. PREVENTIVE SERVICES TASK FORCE RECOMMENDATION

Population	All newborn infants
Recommendation	Screen for hearing loss in all newborn infants. Grade: B
Risk Assessment	The prevalence of hearing loss in newborn infants with specific risk indicators is 10 to 20 times higher than in the general population of newborns. Risk indicators associated with permanent bilateral congenital hearing loss include: • Neonatal intensive care unit admission for 2 or more days. • Family history of hereditary childhood sensorineural hearing loss. • Craniofacial abnormalities. • Certain congenital syndromes and infections. Approximately 50% of newborns with permanent bilateral congenital hearing loss do not have any known risk indicators.
Screening Tests	Screening programs should be conducted using a one-step or two-step validated protocol. A frequently-used 2-step screening process involves otoacoustic emissions followed by auditory brain stem response in newborns who fail the first test. Infants with positive screening tests should receive appropriate audiologic evaluation and follow-up after discharge. Procedures for screening and follow-up should be in place for newborns delivered at home, birthing centers, or hospitals without hearing screening facilities.
Timing of Screening	All infants should have hearing screening before one month of age. Infants who do not pass the newborn screening should undergo audiologic and medical evaluation before 3 months of age.
Treatment	Early intervention services for hearing-impaired infants should meet the individualized needs of the infant and family, including acquisition of communication competence, social skills, emotional well-being, and positive self-esteem. Early intervention comprises evaluation for amplification or sensory devices, surgical and medical evaluation, and communication assessment and therapy. Cochlear implants are usually considered for children with severe-to-profound hearing loss only after inadequate response to hearing aids.
Other Relevant USPSTF Recommendations	Additional USPSTF recommendations regarding screening tests for newborns can be accessed at http://www.uspreventiveservicestaskforce.org/recommendations.htm#pediatric.

For a summary of the evidence systematically reviewed in making these recommendations, the full recommendation statement, and supporting documents, please go to http://www.uspreventiveservicestaskforce.org.

SCREENING OF INFANTS FOR HYPERBILIRUBINEMIA TO PREVENT CHRONIC BILIRUBIN ENCEPHALOPATHY

CLINICAL SUMMARY OF U.S. PREVENTIVE SERVICES TASK FORCE RECOMMENDATION

Population	Healthy newborn infants ≥35 weeks' gestational age
Recommendation	No recommendation. Grade: I (Insufficient Evidence)

Risk Assessment	Risk factors for hyperbilirubinemia include family history of neonatal jaundice, exclusive breastfeeding, bruising, cephalohematoma, ethnicity (Asian, black), maternal age >25 years, male gender, G6PD deficiency, and gestational age <36 weeks. The specific contribution of these risk factors to chronic bilirubin encephalopathy in healthy children is not well understood.
Importance	Chronic bilirubin encephalopathy is a rare but devastating condition. Not all children with chronic bilirubin encephalopathy have a history of hyperbilirubinemia.
Balance of Benefits and Harms	Evidence about the benefits and harms of screening is lacking. Therefore, the USPSTF could not determine the balance of benefits and harms of screening newborns for hyperbilirubinemia to prevent chronic bilirubin encephalopathy.
Considerations for Practice	In deciding whether to screen, clinicians should consider the following: • **Potential preventable burden.** Bilirubin encephalopathy is a relatively rare disorder. Hyperbilirubinemia alone does not account for the neurologic condition of chronic bilirubin encephalopathy. There is no known screening test that will reliably identify all infants at risk of developing chronic bilirubin encephalopathy. • **Potential harms.** Potential harms of screening are unmeasured but may be important. Evidence about the potential harms of phototherapy is lacking. Harms of treatment by exchange transfusion may include apnea, bradycardia, cyanosis, vasospasm, thrombosis, necrotizing enterocolitis, and, rarely, death. • **Current practice.** Universal screening is widespread in the United States.
Screening Tests	Screening may consist of risk-factor assessment, measurement of bilirubin level either in serum or by transcutaneous estimation, or a combination of methods.
Interventions	Phototherapy is commonly used to treat hyperbilirubinemia. Exchange transfusion is used to treat extreme hyperbilirubinemia.
Relevant USPSTF Recommendations	USPSTF recommendations on screening newborns for hearing loss, congenital hypothyroidism, hemoglobinopathies, and phenylketonuria (PKU) can be found at http://www.uspreventiveservicestaskforce.org.

For a summary of the evidence systematically reviewed in making these recommendations, the full recommendation statement, and supporting documents, please go to http://www.uspreventiveservicestaskforce.org.

PART I: SCREENING FOR IRON DEFICIENCY ANEMIA IN CHILDREN AND PREGNANT WOMEN

CLINICAL SUMMARY OF U.S. PREVENTIVE SERVICES TASK FORCE RECOMMENDATION

Population	Asymptomatic children ages 6 to 12 months	Asymptomatic pregnant women
Recommendation	No recommendation. Grade: I (Insufficient Evidence)	Screen for iron deficiency anemia. Grade: B
Risk Assessment	Individuals considered to be at high risk for iron deficiency include adult women, recent immigrants, and, among adolescent females, fad dieters, as well as those who are obese. Premature and low birth weight infants are also at increased risk for iron deficiency.	
Screening Tests	Serum hemoglobin or hematocrit is the primary screening test for identifying anemia. Hemoglobin is sensitive for iron deficiency anemia; however, it is not sensitive for iron deficiency because mild deficiency states may not affect hemoglobin levels. Potential harms of screening include false-positive results, anxiety, and cost.	
Interventions	Iron deficiency anemia is usually treated with oral iron preparations. The likelihood that iron deficiency anemia identified by screening will respond to treatment is unclear, because many families do not adhere to treatment and because the rate of spontaneous resolution is high.	
Balance of Benefits and Harms	The USPSTF was unable to determine the balance between the benefits and harms of routine screening for iron deficiency anemia in asymptomatic children ages 6 to 12 months.	The benefits of routine screening for iron deficiency anemia in asymptomatic pregnant women outweigh the potential harms.
Other Relevant USPSTF Recommendations	The USPSTF has also made recommendations on screening for blood lead levels in children and pregnant women. These recommendations are available at http://www.uspreventiveservicestaskforce.org/.	

For a summary of the evidence systematically reviewed in making this recommendation, the full recommendation statement, and supporting documents, please go to http://www.uspreventiveservicestaskforce.org/.

65

PART II: IRON SUPPLEMENTATION FOR CHILDREN AND PREGNANT WOMEN

CLINICAL SUMMARY OF U.S. PREVENTIVE SERVICES TASK FORCE RECOMMENDATION

Population	Asymptomatic children ages 6 to 12 months who are at increased risk for iron deficiency anemia	Asymptomatic children ages 6 to 12 months who are at average risk for iron deficiency anemia	Pregnant women who are not anemic
Recommendation	Provide routine iron supplementation. Grade: B	No recommendation. Grade: I (Insufficient Evidence)	No recommendation. Grade: I (Insufficient Evidence)
Risk Assessment	A validated risk assessment tool to guide primary care physicians in identifying individuals who would benefit from iron supplementation has not been developed.		
Preventive Medication	Iron supplementation, such as iron-fortified formula or iron supplements, may improve neurodevelopmental outcomes in children at increased risk for iron deficiency anemia. There is poor evidence that it improves neurodevelopmental or health outcomes in other populations. Oral iron supplementation increases the risk for unintentional overdose and gastrointestinal symptoms. Given appropriate protection against overdose, these harms are small.		
Balance of Benefits and Harms	The moderate benefits of iron supplementation in asymptomatic children ages 6 to 12 months who are at increased risk for iron deficiency anemia outweigh the potential harms.	The USPSTF was unable to determine the balance between the benefits and harms of iron supplementation in children ages 6 to 12 months who are at average risk for iron deficiency anemia.	The USPSTF was unable to determine the balance between the benefits and harms of iron supplementation in non-anemic pregnant women.
Other Relevant USPSTF Recommendations	The USPSTF has also made recommendations on folic acid supplementation in women planning or capable of pregnancy and vitamin D supplementation to prevent cancer and fractures. These recommendations are available at http://www.uspreventiveservicestaskforce.org/.		

For a summary of the evidence systematically reviewed in making this recommendation, the full recommendation statement, and supporting documents, please go to http://www.uspreventiveservicestaskforce.org/.

SCREENING FOR LIPID DISORDERS IN CHILDREN

CLINICAL SUMMARY OF U.S. PREVENTIVE SERVICES TASK FORCE RECOMMENDATION

Population	Asymptomatic infants, children, adolescents, and young adults (age 20 years or younger)
Recommendation	No recommendation. Grade: I (Insufficient Evidence)

Risk Assessment	Risk factors for dyslipidemia include overweight, diabetes, and a family history of common familial dyslipidemias (e.g., familial hypercholesterolemia).
Screening Tests	Serum lipid (total cholesterol, high-density and low-density lipoprotein cholesterol) levels are accurate screening tests for childhood dyslipidemia, although many children with multifactorial types of dyslipidemia will have normal lipid levels in adulthood. The use of family history as a screening tool for dyslipidemia has variable accuracy, largely because definitions of a positive family history and lipid threshold values vary substantially.
Interventions	The effectiveness of treatment interventions (diet, exercise, lipid-lowering agents) in improving health outcomes in children with dyslipidemia (including multifactorial dyslipidemia) remains a critical research gap. Potential harms of screening may include labeling of children whose dyslipidemia would not persist into adulthood or cause health problems. Adverse effects from lipid-lowering medications and low-fat diets, including potential long-term harms, have been inadequately evaluated in children.
Balance of Benefits and Harms	The USPSTF was unable to determine the balance between the potential benefits and harms of routinely screening children and adolescents for dyslipidemia.
Other Relevant USPSTF Recommendations	The USPSTF has made recommendations on screening for lipid disorders in adults and screening for carotid artery stenosis, coronary heart disease, high blood pressure, and peripheral arterial disease. These recommendations are available at http://www.uspreventiveservicestaskforce.org/.

For a summary of the evidence systematically reviewed in making this recommendation, the full recommendation statement, and supporting documents, please go to http://www.uspreventiveservicestaskforce.org/.

SCREENING AND TREATMENT FOR MAJOR DEPRESSIVE DISORDER IN CHILDREN AND ADOLESCENTS

CLINICAL SUMMARY OF U.S. PREVENTIVE SERVICES TASK FORCE RECOMMENDATION

Population	Adolescents (12-18 years)	Children (7-11 years)
Recommendation	Screen when systems for diagnosis, treatment, and followup are in place. Grade: B	No Recommendation Grade: I (Insufficient Evidence)
Risk Assessment	Risk factors for major depressive disorder (MDD) include parental depression, having comorbid mental health or chronic medical conditions, and having experienced a major negative life event.	
Screening Tests	The following screening tests have been shown to do well in teens in primary care settings: • Patient Health Questionnaire for Adolescents (PHQ-A). • Beck Depression Inventory-Primary Care Version (BDI-PC).	Screening instruments perform less well in younger children.
Treatments	Among pharmacotherapies fluoxetine, a selective serotonin reuptake inhibitor (SSRI), has been found efficacious. However, because of risk of suicidality, SSRIs should be considered only if clinical monitoring is possible. Various modes of psychotherapy, and pharmacotherapy combined with psychotherapy, have been found efficacious.	Evidence on the balance of benefits and harms of treatment of younger children is insufficient for a recommendation.

For a summary of the evidence systematically reviewed in making these recommendations, the full recommendation statement, and supporting documents, please go to http://www.uspreventiveservicestaskforce.org.

SCREENING FOR OBESITY IN CHILDREN AND ADOLESCENTS

CLINICAL SUMMARY OF U.S. PREVENTIVE SERVICES TASK FORCE RECOMMENDATION

Population	Children and adolescents 6 to 18 years of age
Recommendation	Screen children aged 6 years and older for obesity. Offer or refer for intensive counseling and behavioral interventions. Grade: B

Screening Tests	BMI is calculated from the weight in kilograms divided by the square of the height in meters. Height and weight, from which BMI is calculated, are routinely measured during health maintenance visits. BMI percentile can be plotted on a chart or obtained from online calculators. Overweight = age- and gender-specific BMI at ≥85th to 94th percentile Obesity = age- and gender-specific BMI at ≥95th percentile
Timing of Screening	No evidence was found on appropriate screening intervals.
Interventions	Refer patients to comprehensive moderate- to high-intensity programs that include dietary, physical activity, and behavioral counseling components.
Balance of Benefits and Harms	Moderate- to high-intensity programs were found to yield modest weight changes. Limited evidence suggests that these improvements can be sustained over the year after treatment. Harms of screening were judged to be minimal.
Other Relevant USPSTF Recommendations	Recommendations on other pediatric and behavioral counseling topics can be found at http://www.uspreventiveservicestaskforce.org.

For a summary of the evidence systematically reviewed in making these recommendations, the full recommendation statement, and supporting documents, please go to http://www.uspreventiveservicestaskforce.org.

69

SCREENING FOR PHENYLKETONURIA

CLINICAL SUMMARY OF U.S. PREVENTIVE SERVICES TASK FORCE RECOMMENDATION

Population	All newborn infants
Recommendation	Screen for Phenykeltonuria (PKU). Grade: A
Screening Tests	Screening for PKU is mandated in all 50 states. Methods of screening vary. Three main methods are used to screen for PKU in the United States: 1. Guthrie Bacterial Inhibition Assay (BIA) 2. Automated fluorometric assay 3. Tandem mass spectrometry
Timing of Screening	Infants who are tested within the first 24 hours after birth should receive a repeat screening test by 2 weeks of age. Optimal timing of screening for premature infants and infants with illnesses is at or near 7 days of age, but in all cases before discharge from the newborn nursery.
Treatment	It is essential that phenylalanine restrictions be instituted shortly after birth to prevent the neurodevelopmental effects of PKU.
Other Relevant USPSTF Recommendations	Additional USPSTF recommendations regarding screening tests for newborns can be accessed at: http://www.uspreventiveservicestaskforce.org/recommendations.htm#pediatric

For a summary of the evidence systematically reviewed in making these recommendations, the full recommendation statement, and supporting documents, please go to http://www.uspreventiveservicestaskforce.org.

SCREENING FOR IDIOPATHIC SCOLIOSIS IN ADOLESCENTS

CLINICAL SUMMARY OF U.S. PREVENTIVE SERVICES TASK FORCE RECOMMENDATION

Population	Asymptomatic adolescents
Recommendation	Do not screen for idiopathic scoliosis. Grade: D
Screening Tests	There is no evidence that screening asymptomatic adolescents detects idiopathic scoliosis at an earlier stage than detection without screening. Screening for idiopathic scoliosis is usually done by visual inspection of the spine to look for asymmetry of the shoulders, scapulae, and hips. If idiopathic scoliosis is suspected, radiography can be used to confirm the diagnosis and to quantify the degree of curvature.
Timing of Screening	Although routine screening of adolescents for idiopathic scoliosis is not recommended, clinicians should be prepared to evaluate idiopathic scoliosis when it is discovered incidentally or when the adolescent or parent expresses concern about scoliosis.
Interventions	Treatment of idiopathic scoliosis during adolescence leads to health benefits (decreased pain and disability) in only a small proportion of people. Most cases detected through screening will not progress to a clinically significant form of scoliosis.
Balance of Benefits and Harms	Treatment of adolescents with idiopathic scoliosis detected through screening leads to moderate harms, including unnecessary brace wear and unnecessary referral for specialty care. As a result, the harms of screening adolescents for idiopathic scoliosis exceed the potential benefits.
Other Relevant USPSTF Recommendations	The USPSTF has also made recommendations on screening for developmental dysplasia of the hip. These recommendations are available at http://www.uspreventiveservicestaskforce.org/.

For a summary of the evidence systematically reviewed in making this recommendation, the full recommendation statement, and supporting documents, please go to http://www.uspreventiveservicestaskforce.org/.

SCREENING FOR SICKLE CELL DISEASE IN NEWBORNS

CLINICAL SUMMARY OF U.S. PREVENTIVE SERVICES TASK FORCE RECOMMENDATION

Population	All newborn infants
Recommendation	Screen for sickle cell disease. Grade: A
Screening Tests	Screening for sickle cell disease in newborns is mandated in all 50 states and the District of Columbia. In most states, one of these tests is used for the initial screening: • Thin-layer isoelectric focusing (IEF). • High performance liquid chromatography (HPLC). Both IEF and HPLC have extremely high sensitivity and specificity for sickle cell anemia.
Timing of Screening	All newborns should undergo screening regardless of birth setting. Birth attendants should make arrangements for samples to be obtained. The first clinician to see the infant at an office visit should verify screening results. Confirmatory testing should occur no later than 2 months of age.
Treatment	Infants with sickle cell anemia should receive: • Prophylactic penicillin starting by age 2 months. • Pneumococcal immunizations at recommended intervals.
Other Relevant USPSTF Recommendations	Additional USPSTF recommendations regarding screening tests for newborns can be accessed at http://www.uspreventiveservicestaskforce.org/recommendations.htm#vision.

For a summary of the evidence systematically reviewed in making these recommendations, the full recommendation statement, and supporting documents, please go to http://www.uspreventiveservicestaskforce.org.

SCREENING FOR SPEECH AND LANGUAGE DELAY IN PRESCHOOL CHILDREN

CLINICAL SUMMARY OF U.S. PREVENTIVE SERVICES TASK FORCE RECOMMENDATION

Population	Children ages 5 years and younger who have not already been identified as at increased risk for speech and language delays
Recommendation	No recommendation. Grade: I (Insufficient Evidence)

Risk Assessment	The most consistently reported risk factors include a family history of speech and language delay, male sex, and perinatal factors, such as prematurity and low birth-weight. Other risk factors reported less consistently include levels of parental education, specific childhood illnesses, birth order, and larger family size.
Screening Tests	There is insufficient evidence that brief, formal screening instruments that are suitable for use in primary care for assessing speech and language development can accurately identify children who would benefit from further evaluation and intervention.
Balance of Benefits and Harms	The USPSTF could not determine the balance of benefits and harms of using brief, formal screening instruments to screen for speech and language delay in the primary care setting.
Other Relevant USPSTF Recommendations	The USPSTF has also made recommendations on screening for hearing loss in newborns and vision impairment in children ages 1 to 5 years. These recommendations are available at http://www.uspreventiveservicestaskforce.org/.

For a summary of the evidence systematically reviewed in making this recommendation, the full recommendation statement, and supporting documents, please go to http://www.uspreventiveservicestaskforce.org/.

SCREENING FOR VISUAL IMPAIRMENT IN CHILDREN AGES 1 TO 5

CLINICAL SUMMARY OF U.S. PREVENTIVE SERVICES TASK FORCE RECOMMENDATION

Population	Children ages 3 to 5 years	Children younger than 3 years of age
Recommendation	Provide vision screening. Grade: B	No recommendation. Grade: I (Insufficient Evidence)
Screening Tests	Various screening tests are used in primary care to identify visual impairment in children, including: • Visual acuity test • Stereoacuity test • Cover-uncover test • Hirschberg light reflex test • Autorefraction • Photoscreening	
Timing of Screening	No evidence was found regarding appropriate screening intervals.	
Interventions	Primary treatment for amblyopia includes the use of corrective lenses, patching, or atropine therapy of the non-affected eye. Treatment may also consist of a combination of interventions.	
Balance of Benefits and Harms	There is adequate evidence that early treatment of amblyopia in children ages 3 to 5 years leads to improved visual outcomes. There is limited evidence on harms of screening, including psychosocial effects, in children ages 3 years and older. There is inadequate evidence that early treatment of amblyopia in children younger than 3 years of age leads to improved visual outcomes.	
Suggestions for Practice Regarding the I Statement	In deciding whether to refer children younger than 3 years of age for screening, clinicians should consider: • *Potential preventable burden:* screening later in the preschool years seems to be as effective as screening earlier • *Costs:* initial high costs associated with autorefractors and photoscreeners • *Current practice:* typical vision screening includes assessment of visual acuity, strabismus, and stereoacuity; children with positive findings should be referred for a comprehensive ophthalmologist exam	

For a summary of the evidence systematically reviewed in making these recommendations, the full recommendation statement, and supporting documents, please go to http://www.uspreventiveservicestaskforce.org.

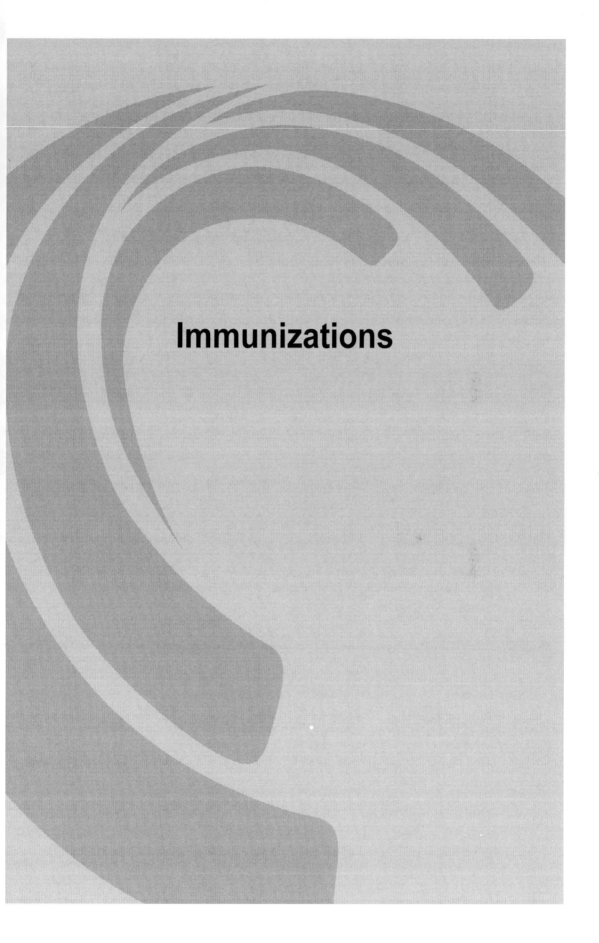

Immunizations

Immunizations for Adults and Children

The USPSTF recognizes the importance of immunizations in primary disease prevention. However, the USPSTF does not wish to duplicate the significant investment of resources made by others to review new evidence on immunizations in a timely fashion and make recommendations.

The Centers for Disease Control and Prevention's (CDC's) Advisory Committee on Immunization Practices (ACIP) publishes recommendations on immunizations for children and adults. The methods used by the ACIP to review evidence on immunizations may differ from the methods used by the USPSTF.

For the ACIP's current recommendations on immunizations, please refer to the National Immunization Program Web site at www.cdc.gov/vaccines/recs/schedules/default.htm.

Topics in Progress

Topics in Progress

Each USPSTF recommendation goes through several stages of development. The review process takes into account input from the medical and research community, stakeholders, and the general public.

The length of time for the entire recommendation process varies depending on the amount and type of available evidence and the time required for compilation of data into a draft recommendation, public comment periods and consideration of comments, and in-depth review and discussions among USPSTF members.

The following topics are in review and are likely to be issued as drafts for public comment during 2012:

- Alcohol Misuse, Screening and Behavioral Counseling
- Breast Cancer, Preventive Medications
- Child Abuse and Neglect, Interventions to Prevent
- Glaucoma, Screening
- Hepatitis C Virus in Adults, Screening
- HIV Infection, Screening
- Thyroid Disease, Screening
- Tobacco Use (Children and Adolescents), Interventions to Prevent

Recommendations on the following topics were published during the production of the *2012 Guide to Clinical Preventive Services* or are in review and are likely to be published as final recommendations during 2012:

- Chronic Kidney Disease, Screening
- Coronary Heart Disease, Screening With Electrocardiography
- Falls in Older Adults, Interventions to Prevent
- Healthful Diet and Physical Activity for CVD Prevention, Counseling
- Hearing Loss in Older Adults, Screening
- Hormone Therapy in Postmenopausal Women, Preventive Medication
- Intimate Partner Violence and Elderly Abuse, Screening
- Obesity in Adults, Screening
- Ovarian Cancer, Screening
- Prostate Cancer, Screening

- Skin Cancer, Counseling
- Vitamin D and Calcium Supplementation to Prevent Cancer and Fractures

The following topics are in earlier stages of review and are likely to be issued as drafts or published as final recommendations sometime after 2012:

- Abdominal Aortic Aneurysm, Screening
- BRCA 1 & 2, Screening and Counseling
- Dementia, Screening
- Gestational Diabetes, Screening
- High Blood Pressure (Children and Adolescents), Screening
- Lung Cancer, Screening
- Oral Cancer, Screening
- Peripheral Artery Disease, Screening
- Suicide Risk, Screening
- Vitamin Supplementation to Prevent Cancer and Cardiovascular Disease

Please visit the USPSTF Recommendations page at www.uspreventiveservices taskforce.org/recommendations.htm to find the most current recommendations, as well as information on the status of topics being updated.

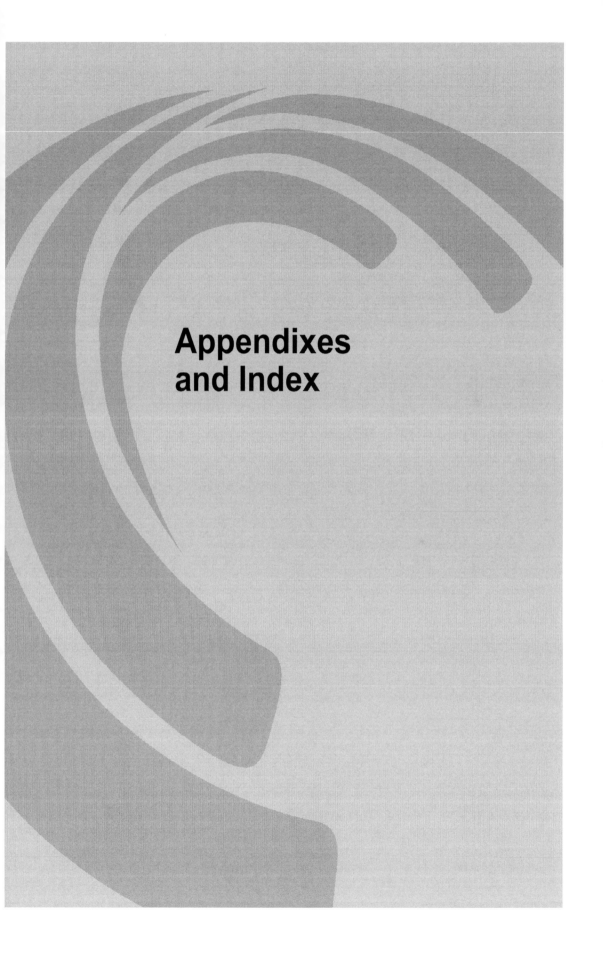

Appendixes
and Index

How the U.S. Preventive Services Task Force Grades Its Recommendations

The U.S. Preventive Services Task Force (USPSTF) assigns one of five letter grades (A, B, C, D, or I) to each of its recommendations to describe the recommendation's strength. In May 2007, the USPSTF changed its grade definitions based on a change in methods and, in July 2012, it updated the definition and suggestions for practice for the grade C recommendations.

Describing the strength of a recommendation is an important part of communicating its importance to clinicians and other users. Although most of the grade definitions have evolved since the Task Force first began, none has changed more noticeably than the definition for a C recommendation, which has undergone three major revisions since 1998. Despite these revisions, the essence of the C recommendation has remained consistent: At the population level, the balance of benefits and harms is very close, and the magnitude of net benefit is small. Given this small net benefit, the Task Force has either: not made a recommendation "for or against routinely" providing the service (1998); recommended "against routinely" providing the service (2007); or recommended "selectively" providing the service (2012). Grade C recommendations are particularly sensitive to patient values and circumstances. Determining whether or not the service should be offered or provided to an individual patient will typically require an informed conversation between clinician and patient.

Grade Definitions After May 2007

What the Grades Mean and Suggestions for Practice

With the USPSTF's 2007 updates to grade definitions, suggestions for practice are now associated with each grade. The USPSTF had also defined levels of certainty regarding net benefit. These definitions apply to USPSTF recommendations voted on or after May 2007.

Grade	Definition	Suggestions for Practice
A	The USPSTF recommends the service. There is high certainty that the net benefit is substantial.	Offer or provide this service.
B	The USPSTF recommends the service. There is high certainty that the net benefit is moderate or there is moderate certainty that the net benefit is moderate to substantial.	Offer or provide this service.
C*	The USPSTF recommends against routinely providing the service. There may be considerations that support providing the service in an individual patient. There is at least moderate certainty that the net benefit is small.	Offer or provide this service only if other considerations support the offering or providing the service in an individual patient.
D	The USPSTF recommends against the service. There is moderate or high certainty that the service has no net benefit or that the harms outweigh the benefits.	Discourage the use of this service.
I Statement	The USPSTF concludes that the current evidence is insufficient to assess the balance of benefits and harms of the service. Evidence is lacking, of poor quality, or conflicting, and the balance of benefits and harms cannot be determined.	Read the clinical considerations section of USPSTF Recommendation Statement. If the service is offered, patients should understand the uncertainty about the balance of benefits and harms.

*The USPSTF voted on the following definition of Grade C in July 2012. The new definition, voted while this Guide was in final production, does not apply to any of the recommendations in this Guide. *Grade Definition:* The USPSTF recommends selectively offering (or providing) this service to individual patients based on professional judgment and patient preferences. There is at least moderate certainty that the net benefit is small. *Suggestions for Practice:* Offer or provide this service for selected patients depending on individual circumstances.

Levels of Certainty Regarding Net Benefit

Level of Certainty*	Description
High	The available evidence usually includes consistent results from well-designed, well-conducted studies in representative primary care populations. These studies assess the effects of the preventive service on health outcomes. This conclusion is therefore unlikely to be strongly affected by the results of future studies.
Moderate	The available evidence is sufficient to determine the effects of the preventive service on health outcomes, but confidence in the estimate is constrained by such factors as: • The number, size, or quality of individual studies. • Inconsistency of findings across individual studies. • Limited generalizability of findings to routine primary care practice. • Lack of coherence in the chain of evidence. As more information becomes available, the magnitude or direction of the observed effect could change, and this change may be large enough to alter the conclusion.
Low	The available evidence is insufficient to assess effects on health outcomes. Evidence is insufficient because of: • The limited number or size of studies. • Important flaws in study design or methods. • Inconsistency of findings across individual studies. • Gaps in the chain of evidence. • Findings not generalizable to routine primary care practice. • Lack of information on important health outcomes. More information may allow estimation of effects on health outcomes.

*The USPSTF defines certainty as "likelihood that the USPSTF assessment of the net benefit of a preventive service is correct." The net benefit is defined as benefit minus harm of the preventive service as implemented in a general, primary care population. The USPSTF assigns a certainty level based on the nature of the overall evidence available to assess the net benefit of a preventive service.

Grade Definitions Prior to May 2007

The definitions below (of USPSTF grades and quality of evidence ratings) were in use prior to the update and apply to recommendations voted on by the USPSTF prior to May 2007.

A — Strongly Recommended: The USPSTF strongly recommends that clinicians provide [the service] to eligible patients. The USPSTF found good evidence that [the service] improves important health outcomes and concludes that benefits substantially outweigh harms.

B — Recommended: The USPSTF recommends that clinicians provide [the service] to eligible patients. The USPSTF found at least fair evidence that [the service] improves important health outcomes and concludes that benefits outweigh harms.

C — No Recommendation: The USPSTF makes no recommendation for or against routine provision of [the service]. The USPSTF found at least fair evidence that [the service] can improve health outcomes but concludes that the balance of benefits and harms is too close to justify a general recommendation.

D — Not Recommended: The USPSTF recommends against routinely providing [the service] to asymptomatic patients. The USPSTF found at least fair evidence that [the service] is ineffective or that harms outweigh benefits.

I — Insufficient Evidence to Make a Recommendation: The USPSTF concludes that the evidence is insufficient to recommend for or against routinely providing [the service]. Evidence that [the service] is effective is lacking, of poor quality, or conflicting and the balance of benefits and harms cannot be determined.

Quality of Evidence

The USPSTF grades the quality of the overall evidence for a service on a 3-point scale (good, fair, poor):

Good: Evidence includes consistent results from well-designed, well-conducted studies in representative populations that directly assess effects on health outcomes.

Fair: Evidence is sufficient to determine effects on health outcomes, but the strength of the evidence is limited by the number, quality, or consistency of the individual studies, generalizability to routine practice, or indirect nature of the evidence on health outcomes.

Poor: Evidence is insufficient to assess the effects on health outcomes because of limited number or power of studies, important flaws in their design or conduct, gaps in the chain of evidence, or lack of information on important health outcomes.

Appendix B

Members of the U.S. Preventive Services Task Force 2002-2012

Janet D. Allan, Ph.D., R.N., C.S., F.A.A.N.
School of Nursing
University of Maryland, Baltimore
Baltimore, MD

Linda Ciofu Baumann, Ph.D., R.N.
School of Nursing and School of
    Medicine & Public Health
University of Wisconsin
Madison, WI

Alfred O. Berg, M.D., M.P.H.
University of Washington
Seattle, WA

Kirsten Bibbins-Domingo, Ph.D., M.D.
San Francisco General Hospital
University of California,
San Francisco, CA

Adelita Gonzales Cantu, R.N., Ph.D.
University of Texas Health Science
    Center
San Antonio, TX

Ned Calonge, M.D., M.P.H.
Colorado Department of Public Health
    and Environment
Denver, CO

Susan J. Curry, Ph.D.
College of Public Health
University of Iowa
Iowa City, IA

Thomas G. DeWitt, M.D.
Department of Pediatrics
Children's Hospital Medical Center
Cincinnati, OH

Allen J. Dietrich, M.D.
Dartmouth Medical School
Hanover, NH

Mark Ebell, M.D., M.S.
The University of Georgia
Athens, GA

Glenn Flores, M.D.
University of Texas
Southwestern Medical Center and
    Children's Medical Center of Dallas
Dallas, TX

Paul S. Frame, M.D.
Tri-County Family Medicine
Cohocton, MY

Joxel Garcia, M.D., M.B.A.
Pan American Health Organization
Washington, DC

Leon Gordis, M.D., Dr.P.H.
Johns Hopkins Bloomberg School of
    Public Health
Baltimore, MD

Kimberly D. Gregory, M.D., M.P.H.
Cedars-Sinai Medical Center
Los Angeles, CA

David Grossman, M.D., M.P.H.
Center for Health Studies, Group
    Health Cooperative
University of Washington
Seattle, WA

Russell Harris, M.D., M.P.H.
University of North Carolina School of
    Medicine
Chapel Hill, NC

Jessica Herzstein, M.D., M.P.H.
Air Products
Allentown, PA

Charles J. Homer, M.D., M.P.H.
National Initiative for Children's
Healthcare Quality
Boston, MA

George Isham, M.D., M.S.
HealthPartners
Minneapolis, MN

Mark S. Johnson, M.D., M.P.H.
New Jersey Medical School
University of Medicine and Dentistry of
New Jersey
Newark, NJ

Kenneth Kizer, M.D., M.P.H.
National Quality Forum
Washington, DC

Jonathan D. Klein, M.D., M.P.H.
University of Rochester
Rochester, NY

Tracy A. Lieu, M.D., M.P.H.
Harvard Pilgrim Health Care and
Harvard Medical School
Boston, MA

Michael L. LeFevre, M.D., M.S.P.H.
University of Missouri School of
Medicine
Columbia, MO

Rosanne Leipzig, M.D., Ph.D.
Mount Sinai School of Medicine
New York, NY

Carol Loveland-Cherry, Ph.D., R.N.,
F.A.A.N.
School of Nursing
University of Michigan
Ann Arbor, MI

Lucy N. Marion, Ph.D., R.N.
School of Nursing
Medical College of Georgia
Augusta, GA

Joy Melnikow, M.D., M.P.H.
University of California Davis
Sacramento, CA

Bernadette Melnyk, Ph.D., R.N.,
C.P.N.P./N.P.P.
College of Nursing & Healthcare
Innovation
Arizona State University
Phoenix, AZ

Virginia A. Moyer, M.D., M.P.H.
University of Texas Health Science
Center
Houston, TX

Cynthia D. Mulrow, M.D., M.Sc.
University of Texas Health Science
Center
Audie L. Murphy Memorial Veterans
Hospital
San Antonio, TX

Wanda Nicholson, M.D., M.P.H.,
M.B.A.
Johns Hopkins School of Medicine and
Bloomberg School of Public Health
Baltimore, MD

Judith K. Ockene, Ph.D., M.Ed.
University of Massachusetts Medical
School
Worcester, MA

C. Tracy Orleans, Ph.D.
The Robert Wood Johnson Foundation
Princeton, NJ

Douglas K. Owens, M.D., M.S.
VA Palo Alto Health Care System
Freeman Spogli Institute for
    International Studies
Stanford University
Stanford, CA

Jeffrey F. Peipert, M.D., M.P.H.
Women and Infants' Hospital
Providence, RI

Nola J. Pender, Ph.D., R.N.
School of Nursing
University of Michigan
Ann Arbor, MI

Diana B. Petitti, M.D., M.P.H.
Fulton School of Engineering
Arizona State University
Tempe, AZ

Carolina Reyes, M.D.
University of Southern California,
    Los Angeles County/USC Medical
    Center
Los Angeles, CA

George F. Sawaya, M.D.
University of California, San Francisco
San Francisco, CA

J. Sanford (Sandy) Schwartz, M.D.
University of Pennsylvania School of
    Medicine and Wharton School
Philadelphia, PA

Harold C. Sox, Jr., M.D.
Dartmouth-Hitchcock Medical Center
Lebanon, NH

Albert L. Siu, M.D.
Mount Sinai Medical Center
New York, NY

Steven M. Teutsch, M.D., M.P.H.
Merck and Company, Inc.
West Point, PA

Carolyn Westhoff, M.D., M.Sc.
Columbia University
New York, NY

Timothy Wilt, M.D., M.P.H.
Minneapolis VA Medical Center
University of Minnesota
Minneapolis, MN

Steven H. Woolf, M.D., M.P.H.
Virginia Commonwealth University
Fairfax, VA

**Barbara P. Yawn, M.D., M.S.P.H.,
    M.Sc.**
Olmstead Medical Center
Rochester, MN

Appendix C

Acknowledgements

AHRQ Staff Supporting the USPSTF 2012

Aileen Buckler, M.D., M.P.H.
Joel Boches
Robert Cosby, Ph.D.
Jennifer Croswell, M.D., M.P.H.
Sandra K. Cummings
Farah Englert
Saeed Fatemi
Janice Genevro, Ph.D., M.S.W.
Margi Grady
Alison Hunt
William Hyde, M.L.S.
Kristie Kiser
Biff LeVee
Iris Mabry-Hernandez, M.D., M.P.H.
Corey Mackison, M.S.A.
Andrew Marshall
Robert McNellis, M.P.H., P.A.
David Meyers, M.D.
Tess Miller, Dr.P.H.
Emily Moser
Lisa Nicolella
Linwood Norman, M.S.
Janine Payne, M.P.H.
Kathryn Ramage
Richard Ricciardi, Ph.D., N.P., F.A.A.N.P.
Randie Siegel, M.S.
Gloria Washington
Rachel Weinstein
Claire Weschler, M.S.Ed.
Tracy Wolff, M.D., M.P.H.

Evidence-Based Practice Centers Supporting the USPSTF for Recommendations in the 2012 Edition

The following researchers, working through four AHRQ Evidence-Based Practice Centers, prepared systematic evidence reviews and evidence summaries as resources on topics under consideration by the USPSTF.

Oregon Evidence-Based Practice Center:

Howard Balshem, M.S.; Tracy Beil, M.S.; Ian Blazina, M.P.H.; Christina Bougatsos, M.P.H.; Brittany Burda, M.P.H.; Amy Cantor, M.D., M.P.H.; Roger Chou, M.D.; Erika Cottrell, Ph.D., M.P.P.; Tracy Dana, M.L.S.; Mark Deffebach, M.D.; Elizabeth Eckstrom, M.D.; Michelle Eder, Ph.D.; Stephen Fortmann, M.D.; Rochelle Fu, Ph.D.; Jessica Griffin, M.A.; Jeanne-Marie Guise, M.D., M.P.H.; Andrew Hamilton, M.S., M.L.S.; Mark Helfand, M.D., M.P.H.; Linda Humphrey, M.D., M.P.H.; Tanya Kapka, M.D., M.P.H.; P. Todd Korthuis, M.D., M.P.H; Jennifer Lin, M.D.; Kevin W. Lutz, M.F.A.; Yvonne Michael, Sc.D.; Jennifer Mitchell, B.A.; Heidi D. Nelson, M.D., M.P.H.; Carrie Patnode, Ph.D., M.P.H.; Leslie Perdue, M.P.H; Daphne Plaut, M.L.S.; Elizabeth O'Connor, Ph.D.; Basmah Rahman, M.P.H.; Bruin Rugge, M.D., M.P.H.; Shelley Selph, M.D.; Caitlyn Senger, M.P.H.; Christopher Slatore, M.D., M.E.; Beth Smith, D.O.; Xin Sun, Ph.D.; Matthew Thompson, M.D., M.P.H., D.Phil.; Kimberly Vesco, M.D., M.P.H.; Miranda Walker, M.A.; Ngoc Wasson, M.P.H.; Evelyn P. Whitlock, M.D., M.P.H.; Clara Williams, M.P.A.; Bernadette Zakher, M.B.B.S.

RTI International/University of North Carolina Evidence-Based Practice Center

Alice Ammerman, Dr.P.H., R.D.; James D. Bader, D.D.S., M.P.H.; Rainer Beck, M.D.; John F. Boggess, M.D.; Malaz Boustani, M.D., M.P.H.; Seth Brody, M.D.; Audrina J. Bunton; Katrina Donahue, M.D., M.P.H.; Louise Fernandez, P.A.-C., R.D., M.P.H.; Kenneth Fink, M.D., M.G.A., M.P.H.; Carol Ford, M.D.; Angela Fowler-Brown, M.D.; Bradley N. Gaynes, M.D., M.P.H.; Paul Godley, M.D., M.P.H.; Susan A. Hall, M.S.; Laura Hanson, M.D., M.P.H.; Russell Harris, M.D., M.P.H.; Katherine E.Hartmann, M.D., Ph.D.; Michael Hayden, M.D.; M. Brian Hemphill, M.D.; Alissa Driscoll Jacobs, M.S., R.D.; Jana Johnson; Linda Kinsinger, M.D., M.P.H.; Carol Krasnov; Ramesh Krishnaraj; Carole M. Lannon, M.D., M.P.H.; Carmen Lewis, M.D., M.P.H.; Kathleen N. Lohr, Ph.D.; Linda J. Lux, M.P.A.; Kathleen McTigue, M.D., M.P.H.; Catherine Mills, M.A.; Kavita Nanda, M.D., M.H.S.; Carla Nester, M.D.; Britt Peterson, M.D., M.P.H.; Christopher J. Phillips, M.D., M.P.H.; Michael Pignone, M.D., M.P.H.; Mark Pletcher, M.D., M.P.H.; Saif S. Rathore; Melissa Rich, M.D.; Gary Rozier, D.D.S.; Jerry L. Rushton, M.D., M.P.H.; Lucy A. Savitz; Joe Scattoloni; Stacey Sheridan, M.D., M.P.H.; Sonya Sutton, B.S.P.H.; Jeffrey A. Tice, M.D.; Suzanne L. West, Ph.D.; B. Lynn Whitener, Dr.P.H., M.S.L.S.; Margaret Wooddell, M.A.; Dennis Zolnoun, M.D.

University of Ottawa Evidence-Based Practice Center
Nicholas Barrowman, Ph.D.; Catherine Code, M.D., F.R.C.P.C.; Catherine Dubé,
M.D., M.Sc., F.R.C.P.C.; Gabriela Lewin, M.D.; David Moher, Ph.D.; Alaa Rostom,
M.D., M.Sc., F.R.C.P.C.; Margaret Sampson, M.I.L.S.; Alexander Tsertsvadze, M.D.,
M.Sc.

Tufts - New England Medical Center Evidence-Based Practice Center
Priscilla Chew; Mei Chung, Ph.D., M.P.H.; Deirdre DeVine; Stanley Ip, M.D.;
Joseph Lau, M.D.; Gowri Raman, M.D.; Thomas Trikalinos, M.D., Ph.D.

Liaisons to the USPSTF

Primary care partners include:

- American Academy of Family Physicians (AAFP)
- American Academy of Nurse Practitioners (AANP)
- American Academy of Pediatrics (AAP)
- American Academy of Physician Assistants (AAPA)
- American College of Obstetricians and Gynecologists (ACOG)
- American College of Physicians (ACP)
- American College of Preventive Medicine (ACPM)
- American Osteopathic Association (AOA)
- National Association of Pediatric Nurse Practitioners (NAPNAP)

Policy, population, and quality improvement partners include:

- America's Health Insurance Plans (AHIP)
- AARP
- National Committee for Quality Assurance (NCQA)

Federal partners include:

- Centers for Disease Control and Prevention (CDC)
- Centers for Medicare & Medicaid Services (CMS)
- U.S. Food and Drug Administration (FDA)
- Health Resources and Services Administration (HRSA)
- Indian Health Service (IHS)
- National Institutes of Health (NIH)
- Veteran's Health Administration (VHA)
- Department of Defense/Military Health System (DoD/MHS)
- Office of Disease Prevention and Health Promotion (ODPHP)
- Office of the Surgeon General

About the U.S. Preventive Services Task Force

Overview

Created in 1984, the U.S. Preventive Services Task Force (USPSTF) is an independent group of national experts in prevention and evidence-based medicine that works to improve the health of all Americans by making evidence-based recommendations about clinical preventive services such as:

- Screenings
- Counseling services
- Preventive medications

The Task Force is made up of 16 volunteer members who serve 4-year terms. Members come from the fields of preventive medicine and primary care, including internal medicine, family medicine, pediatrics, behavioral health, obstetrics and gynecology, and nursing. The Task Force is led by a chair and two vice-chairs. Members are appointed by the Director of AHRQ. Members must have no substantial conflicts of interest that could impair the integrity of the work of the Task Force. A list of current USPSTF members, including their biographical information, can be found on the USPSTF Web site (www.USPreventiveServicesTaskForce.org).

Since 1998, through acts of the U.S. Congress, the Agency for Healthcare Research and Quality (AHRQ) has been authorized to convene the Task Force and to provide ongoing scientific, administrative, and dissemination support to the Task Force.

Recommendations

The Task Force makes recommendations to help primary care clinicians and patients decide together whether a preventive service is right for a patient's needs. Its recommendations apply to people who have no signs or symptoms of the specific disease or condition to which a recommendation applies and are for services prescribed, ordered, or delivered in the primary care setting.

Task Force recommendations are based on a rigorous review of existing peer-reviewed evidence. The Task Force assesses the effectiveness of a clinical preventive service by evaluating and balancing the potential benefits and harms of the service. The potential benefits include early identification of disease and improvement in health. The potential harms can include adverse effects of the service itself or inaccurate test results that may lead to additional testing, additional risks or unneeded treatment. The Task Force does not explicitly consider costs in its assessment of the effectiveness of a service. The Task Force assigns each recommendation a letter grade (A, B, C, or D grade or an I statement) based on the strength of the evidence and on the balance of benefits and harms of the preventive service. More information on USPSTF recommendation grades and a list of all current USPSTF recommendations can be found on the USPSTF Web site.

The Recommendation Making Process

The USPSTF is committed to making its work as transparent as possible. As part of this commitment, the Task Force provides opportunities for the public to provide input during each phase of the recommendation process.

The phases of the topic development process are described below and illustrated in "Steps the USPSTF Takes to Make a Recommendation" at the end of this appendix.

Topic Nomination

The USPSTF considers a broad range of clinical preventive services for its recommendations, focusing on screenings, counseling, and preventive medications. Anyone can nominate a topic for consideration by the Task Force.

Research Plan Development

Once the USPSTF selects a topic for review, it works with an Evidence-based Practice Center (EPC) to develop a draft research plan, which guides the recommendation process and includes key questions and target populations. A draft research plan is posted for public comment, and feedback is incorporated into a final research plan.

Evidence Report Development

Using the final research plan as a guide, EPC researchers gather, review, and analyze evidence on the topic and summarize their findings in a detailed evidence report. The evidence report is sent to subject matter experts for review before it is shared with the Task Force. Beginning in 2013, draft evidence reports will also be posted for public comment.

Recommendation Statement Development

Task Force members discuss the evidence report and use the information to determine the effectiveness of a service by weighing the benefits and harms. The USPSTF creates a draft recommendation based on this discussion. The Task Force posts its draft recommendations for public comment and solicits feedback from national stakeholder organizations. All comments are reviewed by the Task Force and used to inform the development of the final recommendation statement.

Final Recommendation Statement

After the public comment period, the USPSTF finalizes the recommendation statement. The final recommendation statement is posted on the USPSTF Web site along with supporting materials and is also published in a peer-reviewed scientific journal.

Please visit the Task Force Web site (www.USPreventiveServicesTaskForce.org) to learn how and when to nominate topics for consideration by the Task Force or to comment on topics in development.

Online Resources

On the Task Force Web site, people can:

- View all current USPSTF recommendations and supporting materials.

- Learn more about the Task Force methods and processes.

- Nominate a new USPSTF member or a topic for a consideration by the Task Force.

- Provide input on specific draft materials during public comment periods.

- Sign up for the USPSTF listserv to receive USPSTF updates.

- Access the Electronic Preventive Services Selector (ePSS), a quick hands-on tool designed to help primary care clinicians and health care teams identify, prioritize, and offer the screening, counseling, and preventive medication services that are appropriate for their patients. The ePSS is available on the Web (epss.ahrq.gov) or as a mobile phone or PDA application.

- Access MyHealthfinder. MyHealthfinder is a tool for consumers that provides personalized recommendations for preventive services based on the U.S. Preventive Services Task Force; the *Bright Futures* Guidelines; the Centers for Disease Control and Prevention's Advisory Committee on Immunization Practices (ACIP); and the Institute of Medicine's (IOM's) Committee on Preventive Services for Women.

Steps the USPSTF Takes to Make a Recommendation

Create Research Plan

Draft Research Plan
Task Force members work with
Research Plan that guides the
recommendation process.

Invite Public Comments
The draft Research Plan is posted on the USPSTF Web site for public comment.

Finalize Research Plan
The Task Force and EPC make
Final Research Plan.

Compile Evidence Report

Draft Evidence Report
Using the final Research Plan, the
research team at the EPC independently
Report is critiqued by external national
subject matter experts.

Invite Public Comments
(Beginning in 2013)
The draft Evidence Report is posted on the USPSTF Web site for public comment.

Finalize Evidence Report

Develop Recommendation

Draft Recommendation
Task Force members discuss the
create a draft Recommendation.

Invite Public Comments
The draft Recommendation is posted on the USPSTF Web site for public comment. (The Evidence Report is updated and published.)

Finalize Recommendation
The Task Force reviews all
ratify the final Recommendation.

Disseminate Recommendation

Publish and Disseminate Final Recommendation
The final Recommendation and supporting materials are posted on the USPSTF Web site at www.uspreventiveservicestaskforce.org. Final Recommendations also are made available through electronic tools, peer-reviewed journals, and consumer guides.

99

Appendix E

More Resources

 ### AHRQ's Prevention and Chronic Care Program

AHRQ's Prevention and Chronic Care Program Web site (www. preventiveservices.ahrq.gov) presents information that supports AHRQ's mission to improve the quality, safety, efficiency, and effectiveness of health care for all Americans with a focus on evidence-based preventive and chronic care services. The Program's Web site includes tools, resources, and materials to support health care organizations and engage the entire health care delivery system.

The Program includes two overall project areas with specific areas of focus:

- Improving Primary Care Practice
  - Care coordination
  - Clinical-community linkages
  - Health care/system redesign
  - Health information technology integration
  - Behavioral and mental health
  - Self-management support
- Evidence-Based Decisionmaking
  - Clinical decision support
  - Multiple chronic conditions

 ### myhealthfinder

A consumer-friendly resource, myhealthfinder (available at www. healthfinder.gov) helps people create a customized list of relevant recommendations for preventive services based on age, sex, and pregnancy status, along with explanations of each recommendation in plain language.

Stay Healthy Brochures

Consumers can use the information in this series of brochures to learn which screening tests they need and when to get them, which medicines may prevent diseases, and daily steps to take for good health. The series includes *Men Stay Healthy at Any Age, Women Stay Healthy at Any Age, Men Stay Healthy at 50+* and *Women Stay Healthy at 50+*, all in English and Spanish. Go to www.ahrq.gov/clinic/ppipix.htm for the list and choose the title you are interested in.

 Community Preventive Services Task Force:

Established in 1996 by the U.S. Department of Health and Human Services, the Community Preventive Services Task Force (CPSTF) complements the work of the USPSTF, by addressing preventive services at the community level. The CPSTF assists agencies, organizations, and individuals at all levels (national, State, community, school, worksite, and health care system) by providing evidence-based recommendations about community prevention programs and policies that are effective in saving lives, increasing longevity, and improving Americans' quality of life. The recommendations of the CPSTF are available at www. thecommunityguide.org.

 Healthy People 2020

Healthy People 2020 is an initiative from the U.S. Department of Health and Human Services that challenges individuals, communities, and professionals to take specific steps to ensure good health. Healthy People provides science-based, 10-year national objectives for improving the health of all Americans. Read more at www.healthypeople.gov/2020/default.aspx.

 National Guideline Clearinghouse™

A public resource for evidence-based clinical practice guidelines, NGC (guideline.gov/index.aspx) was originally created by AHRQ in partnership with the American Medical Association and the American Association of Health Plans (now America's Health Insurance Plans). The NGC mission is to provide physicians and other health professionals, health care providers, health plans, integrated delivery systems, purchasers, and others an accessible mechanism for obtaining objective, detailed information on clinical practice guidelines and to further their dissemination, implementation, and use of this information.

Canadian Task Force on Preventive Health Care

The Task Force was established by the Public Health Agency of Canada to develop clinical practice guidelines that support primary care providers in delivering preventive health care. The mandate of the Task Force is to develop and disseminate clinical practice guidelines for primary and preventive care, based on systematic analysis of scientific evidence. Read more at www.canadiantaskforce.ca/.

Cancer Control P.L.A.N.E.T.

A service of the National Cancer Institute, the Cancer Control P.L.A.N.E.T. portal provides access to Web-based resources that can help planners, program staff, and researchers to design, implement, and evaluate evidence-based cancer control programs. Read more at cancercontrolplanet.cancer.gov/index.html.

HealthCare.gov

This Web site (www.healthcare.gov), managed by the U.S. Department of Health and Human Services, helps people take health care into their own hands. It provides information about insurance options, using insurance, the Affordable Care Act, comparing providers, and prevention and wellness—including which preventive services are covered under the Act.

SCREENING FOR BREAST CANCER

CLINICAL SUMMARY OF 2002 U.S. PREVENTIVE SERVICES TASK FORCE RECOMMENDATION*

Population	Women ages 40 years and older		
Screening Test	Mammography, with or without clinical breast examination	Clinical breast examination alone	Breast self-examination alone
Recommendation	Screen every 1 to 2 years. Grade: B	No recommendation. Grade: I (Insufficient Evidence)	No recommendation. Grade: I (Insufficient Evidence)
Risk Assessment	Women who are at increased risk for breast cancer (e.g., those with a family history of breast cancer in a mother or sister, a previous breast biopsy revealing atypical hyperplasia, or first childbirth after age 30) are more likely to benefit from regular mammography than women at lower risk.		
Screening Tests	There is fair evidence that mammography screening every 12 to 33 months significantly reduces mortality from breast cancer. Evidence is strongest for women ages 50 to 69 years. For women ages 40 to 49 years, the evidence that screening mammography reduces mortality from breast cancer is weaker, and the absolute benefit of mammography is smaller, than it is for older women. Clinicians should refer patients to mammography screening centers with proper accreditation and quality assurance standards to ensure accurate imaging and radiographic interpretation. Clinicians should adopt office systems to ensure timely and adequate follow-up of abnormal results.		
Balance of Benefits and Harms	The precise age at which the benefits from screening mammography justify the potential harms is a subjective judgment and should take into account patient preferences. Clinicians should inform women about the potential benefits (reduced chance of dying from breast cancer), potential harms (false-positive results, unnecessary biopsies), and limitations of the test that apply to women their age. The balance of benefits and potential harms of mammography improves with increasing age for women ages 40 to 70 years. Clinicians who advise women to perform breast self-examination or who perform routine clinical breast examination to screen for breast cancer should understand that there is currently insufficient evidence to determine whether these practices affect breast cancer mortality, and that they are likely to increase the incidence of clinical assessments and biopsies.		
Other Relevant USPSTF Recommendations	The USPSTF has made recommendations on screening for genetic susceptibility for breast cancer and chemoprevention of breast cancer. These recommendations are available at http://www.uspreventiveservicestaskforce.org/.		

*The U.S. Department of Health and Human Services, in implementing the Affordable Care Act, under the standard it sets out in revised Section 2713(a)(5) of the Public Health Service Act, utilizes the 2002 recommendation on breast cancer screening of the U.S. Preventive Services Task Force.

For a summary of the evidence systematically reviewed in making this recommendation, the full recommendation statement, and supporting documents, please go to http://www.uspreventiveservicestaskforce.org/.

Index

5-A Approach (see Alcohol Misuse, Screening and Behavioral Counseling)

AAA (see Abdominal Aortic Aneurysm, Screening)

Abdominal Aortic Aneurysm, Screening. 7, 82

Alcohol, Avoidance While Driving (see Motor Vehicle Occupant Restraints, Counseling)

Alcohol Misuse, Screening and Behavioral Counseling 8, 81

Anemia, Iron Deficiency (see Iron Deficiency Anemia, Screening)

Ankle Brachial Index (see Peripheral Arterial Disease, Screening)

Aspirin for the Prevention of Cardiovascular Disease, Preventive Medication 9

Aspirin or Nonsteroidal Anti-inflammatory Drugs for Prevention of Colorectal Cancer, Preventive Medication 10

Asymptomatic Bacteriuria (see Bacteriuria, Screening)

Autorefraction (see Visual Impairment in Children Ages 1-5, Screening)

Bacterial Vaginosis in Pregnancy, Screening. 11

Bacteriuria, Screening. 12

Basal Cell Cancer (see Skin Cancer, Screening)

***Bladder Cancer, Screening.** 13

Blood Lead Levels in Childhood and Pregnancy, Screening. 59

Blood Pressure, High (see High Blood Pressure in Adults, Screening)

BMI Screening, Children and Adolescents (see Obesity in Children and Adolescents, Screening)

Bone Mineral Density (see Osteoporosis, Screening)

BRCA Mutation Testing (see Breast and Ovarian Cancer, BRCA Testing, Screening)

Breast and Ovarian Cancer, BRCA Testing, Screening 14, 82

Breast Cancer, Screening. 15, 16

Breast Cancer, Preventive Medications 81

Breast Self Examination [BSE] (see Breast Cancer, Screening)

Breastfeeding, Counseling 17

CA-125 Screening for Ovarian Cancer (see Breast and Ovarian Cancer, BRCA Testing, Screening)

Cancer

(see Aspirin or Nonsteroidal Anti-inflammatory Drugs for Prevention of Colorectal Cancer, Preventive Medication)

(see Bladder Cancer, Screening)

(see Breast and Ovarian Cancer, BRCA Testing, Screening)

(see Breast Cancer, Screening)

(see Cervical Cancer, Screening)

(see Colorectal Cancer, Screening)

(see Lung Cancer Screening)

(see Oral Cancer, Screening)

(see Ovarian Cancer, Screening)

(see Pancreatic Cancer, Screening)

(see Skin Cancer, Screening)

(see Testicular Cancer, Screening)

Carotid Artery Stenosis, Screening...18

*Cervical Cancer, Screening...19

Chest X-Ray (see Lung Cancer, Screening)

Child Abuse and Neglect, Interventions to Prevent 81

Chlamydial Infection, Screening...20

Chronic Bilirubin Encephalopathy (see Hyperbilirubinemia in Infants, Screening)

Chronic Kidney Disease, Screening 81

Chronic Obstructive Pulmonary Disease, Screening.....................21

Clinical Breast Examination [CBE] (see Breast Cancer, Screening)

Colonoscopy (see Colorectal Cancer, Screening)

Colorectal Cancer, Aspirin/NSAIDS (see Aspirin or Nonsteroidal Anti-inflammatory Drugs for Prevention of Colorectal Cancer, Preventive Medication)

Colorectal Cancer, Screening 22

Congenital Hypothyroidism, Screening.....................................60

Coronary Heart Disease Prevention (see Aspirin for the Prevention of Cardiovascular Disease)

Coronary Heart Disease (Risk Assessment, Nontraditional Risk Factors), Screening...23

Coronary Heart Disease, Screening With Electrocardiography 81

COPD (see Chronic Obstructive Pulmonary Disease, Screening)

Cover-Uncover Test (see Visual Impairment in Children Ages 1-5, Screening)

Dementia, Screening..82

Depression in Adults, Screening **24**

Depression or Depressive Disorders in Children and Adolescents (see Major Depressive Disorders in Children and Adolescents, Screening)

Developmental Dysplasia of the Hip, Screening...**61**

Diabetes Mellitus, Screening..**25**

Drug Use, Illicit (see Illicit Drug Use, Screening)

Drug Abuse (see Illicit Drug Use, Screening)

Dysplasia, Hip (see Developmental Dysplasia of the Hip, Screening)

Elevated Blood Lead Levels (see Blood Lead Levels in Childhood and Pregnancy, Screening)

Estrogen Therapy (see Hormone Replacement Therapy, Preventive Medication)

Falls in Older Adults, Counseling 81

Fecal Occult Blood Testing [FOBT] (see Colorectal Cancer, Screening)

Folic Acid to Prevent Neural Tube Defects **26**

Genetic Risk Assessment and BRCA Mutation Testing (see Breast and Ovarian Cancer, BRCA Testing, Screening)

Genital Herpes, Screening **27**

Gestational Diabetes Mellitus, Screening..**28, 82**

Glaucoma, Screening **29, 81**

*Gonococcal Ophthalmia Neonatorum, Preventive Medication **62**

Gonorrhea, Screening..**30**

Healthful Diet and Physical Activity, Counseling..81

Hearing Loss in Newborns, Screening **63**

Hearing Loss in Older Adults, Screening 81

Heart Disease (see Coronary Heart Disease, Nontraditional Risk Factors)

Hemochromatosis, Screening **31**

Hepatitis B Virus, Screening..**32**

Hepatitis B Virus in Pregnant Women, Screening..**33**

Hepatitis C Virus in Adults, Screening...**34, 81**

Hereditary Hemochromatosis (see Hemochromatosis, Screening)

Herpes Simplex Virus (see Genital Herpes, Screening)

High Blood Pressure (Adults), Screening..**35**

High Blood Pressure (Children), Screening..82

High Cholesterol (see Lipid Disorders in Adults OR in Children, Screening)

Hip Dysplasia (see Developmental Dysplasia of the Hip, Screening)

HIV Infection, Screening..**36**

Hirschberg Light Reflex Test (see Visual Impairment in Children Ages 1-5, Screening)

Hormone Replacement Therapy, Preventive Medication................................**37, 81**

HPV Testing (see Cervical Cancer, Screening)

HT or HRT (see Hormone Replacement Therapy, Preventive Medication)

Human Immunodeficiency Virus (see HIV Infection, Screening)

Hyperbilirubinemia in Infants, Screening **64**

Hyperlipidemia (see Lipid Disorders in Adults OR in Children, Screening)

Hypertension (see High Blood Pressure, Screening)

Hypothyroidism, Congenital (see Congenital Hypothyroidism, Screening)

Idiopathic Scoliosis (see Scoliosis in Adolescence, Screening)

Illicit Drug Use, Screening..**38**

Impaired Visual Acuity in Older Adults, Screening................................**39**

Intimate Partner Violence and Elderly Abuse, Screening................................81

Iron Deficiency Anemia, Screening..**65, 66**

Iron Supplementation (see Iron Deficiency Anemia, Screening)

Lead Levels in Blood, Elevated (see Blood Lead Levels in Childhood and Pregnancy, Screening)

Lipid Disorders in Adults, Screening..**40**

Lipid Disorders in Children, Screening..**67**

Low Dose Computerized Tomography (see Lung Cancer, Screening)

Lung Cancer, Screening..**41, 82**

Major Depressive Disorder in Children and Adolescents, Screening................**68**

Major Depressive Disorder in Adults (see Depression in Adults, Screening)

Mammography (see Breast Cancer, Screening)

Melanoma (see Skin Cancer, Screening)

Motor Vehicle Occupant Restraints, Counseling **42**

Neural Tube Defects (see Folic Acid to Prevent Neural Tube Defects)

Newborn Hearing Screening (see Hearing Loss (Newborns), Screening)

Non-Steroidal Anti-Inflammatories [NSAIDS] (see Aspirin or NSAIDs for Primary Prevention of Colorectal Cancer, Preventive Medication)

Obesity in Adults, Screening 81

Obesity in Children and Adolescents, Screening **69**

Oral Cancer, Screening **43, 82**

*Osteoporosis, Screening **44**

Ovarian Cancer, Screening **45, 81**

Overweight (see Obesity in Children and Adolescents, Screening)

Pancreatic Cancer, Screening **46**

Pap Smear (see Cervical Cancer, Screening)

Peripheral Arterial Disease, Screening **47, 82**

Phenylketonuria, Screening **70**

Photoscreening (see Visual Impairment in Children Ages 1-5, Screening)

PKU (see Phenylketonuria, Screening)

Postmenopausal Hormone Therapy (see Hormone Replacement Therapy, Preventive Medication)

Progestin Therapy (see Hormone Replacement Therapy, Preventive Medication)

Prostate Cancer, Screening 81

PSA Screening for Prostate Cancer (see Prostate Cancer, Screening)

Rh (D) Incompatibility, Screening **48**

Scoliosis in Adolescents (Idiopathic), Screening **71**

Sexually Transmitted Infections, Counseling **49**

Sickle Cell Disease, Screening **72**

Sigmoidoscopy (see Colorectal Cancer, Screening)

Skin Cancer, Counseling 82

Skin Cancer, Screening **50**

Speech and Language Delay, Screening **73**

Squamous Cell Cancer (see Skin Cancer, Screening)

Smoking Cessation (see Tobacco Use in Adults, Counseling and Interventions)

Spirometry Screening for COPD (see Chronic Obstructive Pulmonary Disease, Screening)

Sputum Cytology (see Lung Cancer, Screening)

Stereoacuity Test (see Visual Impairment in Children Ages 1-5, Screening)

STI or STD

(see Sexually Transmitted Infections, Counseling)

(see Chlamydial Infection, Screening)

(see Gonorrhea, Screening)

(see Genital Herpes Simplex, Screening)

(see HIV Infection, Screening)

(see Syphilis (Pregnant Women), Screening)

Suicide Risk, Screening **51, 82**

Syphilis Infection, Screening **52**

Syphilis (Pregnant Women), Screening **53**

T3 (see Thyroid Disease, Screening)

T4

(see Thyroid Disease, Screening)

(see Congenital Hypothyroidism, Screening)

***Testicular Cancer, Screening** **54**

Thyroid Disease, Screening **55, 81**

Tobacco (Children and Adolescents), Interventions to Prevent 81

Tobacco Use in Adults, Counseling and Interventions **56**

TSH

(see Thyroid Disease, Screening)

(see Congenital Hypothyroidism, Screening)

Ultrasonography (see Abdominal Aortic Aneurysm, Screening)

Urinalysis (see Bladder Cancer, Screening)

Urine Biomarkers (see Bladder Cancer, Screening)

Urine Culture (see Bacteriuria in Adults, Screening)

Urine Cytology (see Bladder Cancer, Screening)

Vaginosis, Bacterial (see Bacterial Vaginosis in Pregnancy, Screening)

Visual Acuity Test (see Visual Impairment in Children Ages 1-5, Screening)

***Visual Impairment in Children Ages 1-5, Screening** **74**

Vitamin D and Calcium Supplementation to Prevent Cancer and Fractures 82

Vitamin Supplementation to Prevent Cancer and Cardiovascular Disease 82

---

*indicates new recommendations released March 2010 to March 2012.

Bold text indicates topic of recommendation.

Italic text indicates topic in progress.

The U.S. Preventive Services Task Force is always interested in making our resources and tools more useful to those implementing the recommendations in primary care, as well as educating health professions students and patients.

We would love to hear how well we are meeting your needs. Please take our 2-minute survey to give us your feedback on the *2012 Guide to Clinical Preventive Services* at https://www.surveymonkey.com/s/ClinicalGuide.

Made in the USA
San Bernardino, CA
11 June 2014